The Global Eye Health Handbook

Anna C S Tan • Marcus Ang
Ralene Sim
Editors

The Global Eye Health Handbook

A Clinical Guide

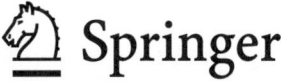

Editors
Anna C S Tan
Department of Medical Retina
Singapore National Eye Centre,
Singapore Eye Research Institute
Singapore, Singapore

Marcus Ang
Department of Cornea and
External Eye
Singapore National Eye Centre,
Singapore Eye Research Institute
Singapore, Singapore

Ralene Sim
Department of Training and
Education
Singapore National Eye Centre,
Singapore Eye Research Institute
Singapore, Singapore

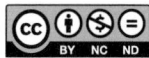

ISBN 978-981-96-8860-9   ISBN 978-981-96-8861-6   (eBook)
https://doi.org/10.1007/978-981-96-8861-6

This work was supported by Singapore Eye Research Institute, Singapore.

© The Editor(s) (if applicable) and The Author(s) 2026. This book is an open access publication.

Open Access This book is licensed under the terms of the Creative Commons Attribution-NonCommercial-NoDerivatives 4.0 International License (http://creativecommons.org/licenses/by-nc-nd/4.0/), which permits any noncommercial use, sharing, distribution and reproduction in any medium or format, as long as you give appropriate credit to the original author(s) and the source, provide a link to the Creative Commons license and indicate if you modified the licensed material. You do not have permission under this license to share adapted material derived from this book or parts of it.

The images or other third party material in this book are included in the book's Creative Commons license, unless indicated otherwise in a credit line to the material. If material is not included in the book's Creative Commons license and your intended use is not permitted by statutory regulation or exceeds the permitted use, you will need to obtain permission directly from the copyright holder.

This work is subject to copyright. All commercial rights are reserved by the author(s), whether the whole or part of the material is concerned, specifically the rights of translation, reprinting, reuse of illustrations, recitation, broadcasting, reproduction on microfilms or in any other physical way, and transmission or information storage and retrieval, electronic adaptation, computer software, or by similar or dissimilar methodology now known or hereafter developed. Regarding these commercial rights a non-exclusive license has been granted to the publisher.

The use of general descriptive names, registered names, trademarks, service marks, etc. in this publication does not imply, even in the absence of a specific statement, that such names are exempt from the relevant protective laws and regulations and therefore free for general use.

The publisher, the authors and the editors are safe to assume that the advice and information in this book are believed to be true and accurate at the date of publication. Neither the publisher nor the authors or the editors give a warranty, expressed or implied, with respect to the material contained herein or for any errors or omissions that may have been made. The publisher remains neutral with regard to jurisdictional claims in published maps and institutional affiliations.

This Springer imprint is published by the registered company Springer Nature Singapore Pte Ltd. The registered company address is: 152 Beach Road, #21-01/04 Gateway East, Singapore 189721, Singapore

If disposing of this product, please recycle the paper.

Preface

The Lancet Global Health Commission on Global Eye Health: vision beyond 2020 reports [1] *"High quality eye health services are not universally delivered; concerted action is needed to improve quality and outcomes, providing effective, efficient, safe, timely, equitable, and people-centred care."* In October 2019, the WHO report on vision executive summary estimated that there are 2.2 billion people with vision impairment (VI) or blindness worldwide and over 1 billion of those have conditions that could be treated or prevented [2]. Hence, in 2023 the Singapore National Eye Centre (SNEC) established our Global Eye Health initiative (SNEC-GEH) with the vision: *"To make high quality, holistic eyecare more equitable and accessible through innovation and the cultivation of a vibrant ecosystem of leadership and capacity building."*

The Asia Pacific region is the most populous continent with increasing rates of blindness and VI due to a rapidly ageing population. It is made of diverse regions with wide disparities between economic development, population demographics, social and cultural advancement, with significant imbalance of high-quality eye care delivery, expertise, and resources [3]. From our experience as collaborative partners in the region, we have identified the need for resources that are practical, relevant, and user-friendly that can be used as a guide by primary and secondary eye health practitioners to improve the quality of eye health delivery in the region.

Our *Global Eye Health Handbook: A Clinical Guide* is a resource that we have designed for both primary and secondary eye care professionals to deliver high quality eye care in their community. Part I is aimed to help eye care professionals diagnose, triage, and treat common ocular conditions in low resource settings. This book contains decision trees for common eye complaints, approach to common and sight-threatening conditions as well as basic first-line treatment strategies and guide for triage to tertiary settings. The chapters provide a systematic approach to the diagnosis and management of various common eye conditions such as refractive error, cataract, endophthalmitis, glaucoma, and retinal conditions. The main aim is to guide clinicians faced with these conditions to derive more accurate diagnoses, initiate early, appropriate management, triage appropriately to provide relevant details, and timely referrals to support further care at the tertiary eye care settings. Eye care delivery is significantly improved with prompt diagnosis and intervention at the first-line primary or secondary care setting, and this will facilitate seamless referral to tertiary settings when necessary. We hope to empower practitioners to provide critical care even in resource-limited environments, ultimately safeguarding vision and preventing long-term complications. Our GEH-tips after each chapter is designed to highlight important takeaway points for each conditions relevant to eye care provision in resource limited settings.

The content for Part I is based on a resource called the SNEC-Ocular Emergency Handbook, which has been previously written, edited, and passed down from generations of SNEC Chief Residents and was a guide for residents to provide first-line eye care at the emergency department settings. We would like to acknowledge all the previous contributors of this resource; the generations of doctors that have worked or are currently working at SNEC. The content has been adapted accordingly for the purposes of this book.

Part IV is a compilation of standard operating protocols from a multi-disciplinary eye care team made of nurses, ophthalmic technicians, and optometrists that we have adapted for this publication. The aim of this section is to outline essential protocols and guidelines to adopt best practices to improve primary and secondary provision of eye health services in various outpatient and surgical settings. They cover important areas of infection control, recommended protocols for doing accurate high-quality biometry and refractions, guidelines for common outpatient procedures for lasers and intravitreal injections and suggestions for conducting audits. Most of these guidelines are originally designed for use at the SNEC, and the GEH tips section will summarize main principles may need to be adapted, edited, and translated for the various target contexts and countries. Strengthening eye care delivery and health systems includes a multi-disciplinary approach and we would like to acknowledge all the SNEC eye care specialists who contributed to the writing and refinement of the content of this section. We hope our target audience with be able to use these valuable resources as a guide to derive their own standard operating procedures to further improve the quality eye care delivery in their communities.

Singapore, Singapore   Anna C S Tan

References

1. Burton MJ, Ramke J, Marques AA, et al. The Lancet Global Health Commission On Global Eye Health: Vision Beyond 2020. *Lancet Glob Health*. Apr 2021;9(4):E489–E551. https://doi.org/10.1016/S2214-109x(20)30488-5
2. *World Report On Vision.* (2019).
3. Yusufu M, Bukhari J, Yu X, Lin TPH, Lam DSC, Wang N. Challenges In Eye Care In The Asia-Pacific Region. *Asia Pac J Ophthalmol (Phila)*. Sept 8 2021;10(5):423–429. https://doi.org/10.1097/Apo.0000000000000391

Disclaimer

This book is intended to serve as a practical guide and reference for clinicians, trainees, and allied eye health professionals. It is not meant to be exhaustive, and readers are encouraged to consult additional sources and current guidelines for comprehensive coverage. While every effort has been made to ensure accuracy, the authors and publishers accept no responsibility for any errors or omissions, nor for any outcomes resulting from the application of information contained herein. Clinical judgment and individualized patient care should always take precedence.

Contents

Part I   A Clinical Guide to Ocular Emergencies and Common Ocular Conditions: Ocular Emergency Flow Charts

1. **Flowcharts: Approach to Blurring of Vision (Mono-ocular)** 3
   Ralene Sim

2. **Flowcharts: Approach to Blurring of Vision (Binocular)** 7
   Ralene Sim

3. **Flowcharts: Approach to Red Eye (Painful)** 11
   Ralene Sim

4. **Flowcharts: Approach to Red Eye (Minimal Pain)** 15
   Ralene Sim

Part II   A Clinical Guide to Ocular Emergencies and Common Ocular Conditions: Ocular Emergencies

5. **Trauma: Corneal Foreign Body** 21
   Yap Guan Hui and Melissa Wong

6. **Trauma: Open Globe Injury** 25
   Yap Guan Hui and Melissa Wong

7	**Trauma: Hyphaema** 31
	Claire Peterson, Zhu Li Yap, and Sahil Thakur
8	**Trauma: Orbital Fracture** 35
	Yap Guan Hui and Yvonne Chung
9	**Trauma: Eyelid Lacerations** 39
	Yap Guan Hui and Yvonne Chung
10	**Trauma: Traumatic Optic Neuropathy (TON)**...... 43
	Reuben Foo, Shweta Singhal, and Umapathi Thirugnanam
11	**Infections: Infective Keratitis**................... 47
	Nicole Sie, Marcus Ang, and Anshu Arundhati
12	**Infections: Conjunctivitis**...................... 53
	Nicole Sie, Marcus Ang, and Anshu Arundhati
13	**Infections: Onchocerciasis** 59
	Nicole Sie, Marcus Ang, and Anshu Arundhati
14	**Infections: Herpes Zoster Ophthalmicus (HZO)**.... 63
	Nicole Sie, Marcus Ang, and Anshu Arundhati
15	**Chemical Injury** 69
	Nicole Sie, Marcus Ang, and Anshu Arundhati
16	**Bullous Keratopathy**........................... 73
	Nicole Sie, Marcus Ang, and Anshu Arundhati
17	**Corneal Graft Rejection**....................... 79
	Nicole Sie and Marcus Ang
18	**Infections: Blebitis** 83
	Claire Peterson, Zhu Li Yap, Sahil Thakur, and Rahat Husain
19	**Infections: Bleb-Related Endophthalmitis** 91
	Claire Peterson, Zhu Li Yap, Sahil Thakur, and Rahat Husain

20	**Acute Angle Closure** .... 95 Claire Peterson, Zhu Li Yap, Sahil Thakur, and Rahat Husain	
21	**Neovascular Glaucoma** .... 99 Claire Peterson, Zhu Li Yap, Sahil Thakur, and Rahat Husain	
22	**Lens-Induced Glaucoma** .... 103 Claire Peterson, Zhu Li Yap, Sahil Thakur, and Shamira Perera	
23	**Acute Anterior Uveitis** .... 107 Joshua Lim and Andrew Tsai	
24	**Infections: Orbital Cellulitis** .... 113 Lim Xian Hui and Yvonne Chung	
25	**Infections: Dacryocystitis** .... 119 Lim Xian Hui and Yvonne Chung	
26	**Carotid Cavernous Fistula (CCF)** .... 123 Reuben Foo, Shweta Singhal, and Umapathi Thirugnanam	
27	**Central Retinal Artery Occlusion (CRAO)**. .... 127 Charles Ong and Anna C S Tan	
28	**Central Retinal Vein Occlusion** .... 131 Charles Ong and Anna C S Tan	
29	**Vitreous Haemorrhage** .... 135 Joshua Lim and Andrew Tsai	
30	**Retinal Detachment** .... 141 Joshua Lim, Andrew Tsai, and Ian Yeo	
31	**Infections: Exogenous (Post-operative) Endophthalmitis** .... 145 Joshua Lim and Andrew Tsai	
32	**Infections: IVT-Related Endophthalmitis** .... 149 Joshua Lim and Andrew Tsai	

33	**Neuro-Ophthalmology: Optic Neuritis** .... 153 Reuben Foo, Shweta Singhal, and Umapathi Thirugnanam	
34	**Neuro-Ophthalmology: Anterior Ischemic Optic Neuropathy (AION)—Arteritic and Non-arteritic.** .... 157 Reuben Foo, Shweta Singhal, and Umapathi Thirugnanam	
35	**Neuro-Ophthalmology: Unilateral Disc Swelling.** ... 163 Reuben Foo, Shweta Singhal, and Umapathi Thirugnanam	
36	**Neuro-Ophthalmology: Bilateral Disc Swelling** ..... 167 Reuben Foo, Shweta Singhal, and Umapathi Thirugnanam	
37	**Diplopia: Oculomotor Palsy (CN3)** .... 173 Reuben Foo, Shweta Singhal, and Umapathi Thirugnanam	
38	**Diplopia: Trochlear Palsy (CN4)** .... 177 Reuben Foo, Shweta Singhal, and Umapathi Thirugnanam	
39	**Diplopia: Abducens Nerve Palsy (CN6)** .... 181 Reuben Foo, Shweta Singhal, and Umapathi Thirugnanam	
40	**Facial Nerve Palsy (CN7)** .... 185 Reuben Foo, Shweta Singhal, and Umapathi Thirugnanam	
41	**Paediatric Emergency: Leukocoria.** .... 189 Lim Sing Hui and Audrey Chia	
42	**Paediatric Emergency: Non-accidental Injury (NAI): Shaken Baby Syndrome** .... 193 Lim Sing Hui and Audrey Chia	
43	**Paediatric Emergency: Allergic Conjunctivitis** ..... 197 Lim Sing Hui and Audrey Chia	

Part III A Clinical Guide to Ocular Emergencies and Common Ocular Conditions: Other Important Conditions and Skills

44 Examination of Paediatric Patients 203
Lim Sing Hui and Audrey Chia

45 A Global Health Approach to Refractive Errors in Children and Adults 207
Bryan Sim and Audrey Chia

46 Cataract 219
Yap Guan Hui and Melissa Wong

47 Age-Related Macular Degeneration 223
Charles Ong and Anna C S Tan

48 Diabetic Retinopathy 229
Charles Ong and Anna C S Tan

49 Central Serous Chorioretinopathy (CSCR) 235
Charles Ong and Anna C S Tan

50 Glaucoma: Referral Pathway 239
Claire Peterson, Zhu Li Yap, Sahil Thakur, and Rahat Husain

Part IV Global Eye Health Protocols and Recommended Standards of Eye Care

51 Hand Hygiene Protocol 245
Low Siew Ngim, Chitra Vallei, and Goh Hui Jin

52 For Nurses 255
Low Siew Ngim, Chitra Vallei, and Goh Hui Jin

53 For Nurses 287
Low Siew Ngim, Chitra Vallei, and Goh Hui Jin

54 Endophthalmitis Prevention 305
Wiryasaputra Shaan and Chitra Vallei

55	**Refraction Protocol**................................ 309
	Kothubutheen Mohamed Farook, Lim Ling Yan, Li Fengxia, and Lim Wei Lan Violet
56	**For Imaging Specialists** 319
	Patrick Ng Yuen Hwa and Hlaing Thandar Aung
57	**Focus on Cataract Outcomes**.................... 341
	Ralene Sim
58	**Introduction to Collecting Audit Data**............. 345
	Ralene Sim

Abbreviations 351

Annexes 355

About the Editors

Anna C S Tan is a Senior Consultant Ophthalmologist at the Singapore National Eye Center and a Clinical Associate Professor at Duke NUS. She is currently the Deputy Head of the Medical Retina Department and the Director of Global Eye Health. Her subspecialty research interests include age-related macular degeneration, diabetic eye disease, low vision, visual rehabilitation, digital technology, and global ophthalmology. She has represented SNEC at many local and international conferences and is a key opinion leader and speaks and sits on multiple advisory boards. She is a successful clinician scientist with over 100 peer-reviewed publications and 4 book chapters and has been the lead editor for the open access *SNEC Global Eye Health Handbook*. She has received multiple competitive grants to further her research interests including the Khoo Clinical Scholarship Award, the Academic Clinical Program Grant for Clinician Scientists, National Medical Council Research Scholarship to pursue her PhD in Clinical Sciences, and recently the Health Services Clinician Scientist Award. She has also won numerous awards such as the Singhealth "Publish" Award in 2020, the "Catalyst Award" in both 2020 and 2021 in US National Academy of Medicines Healthy Longevity Global Competition, the Macula Society Travel Grant in 2021, the Distinguished Service Award in 2022, the ARVO Advocacy Award 2025, and the Pehin Joshi Memorial Teaching Award from the ASEAN Ophthalmology Society in 2025. She is also the treasurer of the Singapore Society of

Ophthalmology and first elected president for the SSO Women's chapter.

Marcus Ang, MBBS, MMED, MCI, FRCS, PhD is Senior Consultant Ophthalmologist and Head of the Cornea and External Eye Disease Service, and Head of Refractive Service, Singapore National Eye Center (SNEC). He also serves as Advisor at the SNEC Myopia Center. He has currently more than 200 peer-reviewed publications (H-index = 57), majority of which are first or corresponding author with JIF>2.0. He has published important peer-reviewed articles in the *LANCET* (IF: 202.7), *LANCET Digital Health* (IF: 36.615), *PRER* (IF: 19.7), *Nature Digital Medicine* (IF: 15.36), and *Ophthalmology* (12.08) and numerous book chapters, including several in the seminal textbook CORNEA. He has more than 20 academic awards, >$5M of competitive research grant funding, and filed 5 patents with 1 licensed. He is a regular invited speaker at international conferences recognized by his international awards such as the APAO Achievement Award (2018) and AAO Achievement Award (2019). As Founding Director of Global Clinic (www.global-clinic.org), he regularly organizes missions and travels to provide free eye-care and cataract surgery in countries such as Indonesia, Thailand, Cambodia, India, and Myanmar. He also serves on the Board of the International Agency for Prevention of Blindness (IAPB) and previously on the Board/Chair of Project Orbis, Singapore. He has been commended with the President's Award for Philanthropy in Singapore (2017), and Outstanding Service in the Prevention of Blindness Award from APAO (2019). He is the current President of the Singapore Society of Ophthalmology. He serves as Secretary of the APAO YO Committee and many regional committees such as the Council for the Asia Pacific Ocular Imaging Society and the Asia Pacific Artificial Cornea and Keraprosthesis Society. As a graduate of the APAO LDP as well as the AAO LDP Class XX, he has contributed to several APAO and AAO committees such as the YO International Committee and AAO Myopia Taskforce. He was recognized with the AAO Secretariat Award in 2021 for his contributions to society work. His contributions and achievements in

Ophthalmology have led to him being awarded the Artemis Award from the American Academy of Ophthalmology in 2019 and Vision Excellence Award (IAPB) in 2020. He has been recognized as one of the Top 100 Ophthalmologists (Global, The Power List 2023 and 2024) and Top 100 Ophthalmologists in the Asia Pacific by the APAO.

Ralene Sim, MBBS, MMed (Ophth), FRCOphth is currently a Senior Resident at the Singapore National Eye Centre. She graduated from the Yong Loo Lin School of Medicine, National University of Singapore, where she was placed on the Dean's List (top 5% of cohort) in 2016 and 2017. She received the SingHealth Medical Student Talent Development Award and Travel Award for her academic and research performance.

Prior to residency, she completed a one-year research fellowship at the Singapore Eye Research Institute, focusing on clinical and translational aspects of ophthalmic research. She has authored multiple first-author publications in leading peer-reviewed journals, presented at international scientific meetings, and received several awards for oral and poster presentations. Her research has also been supported by multiple competitive institutional grants.

She is actively involved in resident education and leadership, serving as Deputy Lead Resident in 2025 and Lead Resident in 2026 for the SingHealth Ophthalmology Residency Programme. She was selected for the SingHealth Junior Educator Development Initiative (JEDI), a program that identifies and supports residents with demonstrated commitment and potential in medical education.

She remains active in community and outreach work, having participated in multiple medical mission trips providing eye and general medical services in underserved regions. She led Project Yangon, an overseas healthcare and education program in Myanmar, as project director (2015–2016), and served on the executive committee of the Neighbourhood Health Service (NHS), a local community health screening initiative.

Part I

A Clinical Guide to Ocular Emergencies and Common Ocular Conditions: Ocular Emergency Flow Charts

Flowcharts: Approach to Blurring of Vision (Mono-ocular)

Ralene Sim

R. Sim (✉)
Department of Training and Education, Singapore National Eye Centre, Singapore Eye Research Institute, Singapore, Singapore
e-mail: ralene.sim@mohh.com.sg

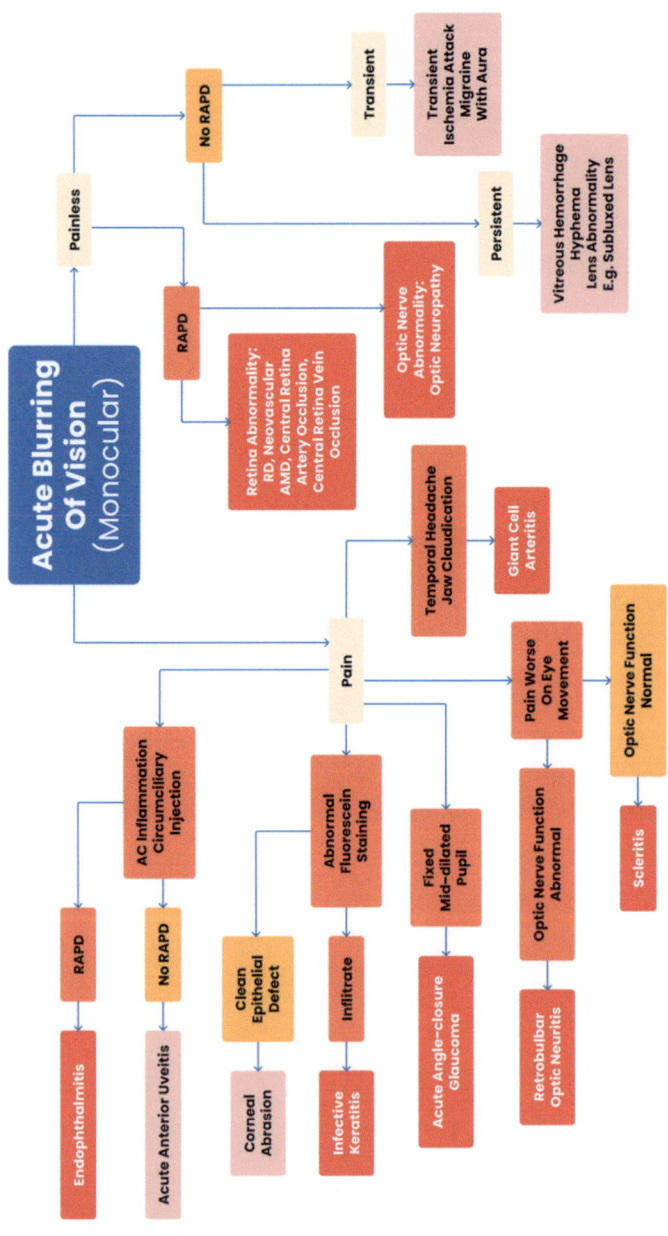

Open Access This chapter is licensed under the terms of the Creative Commons Attribution-NonCommercial-NoDerivatives 4.0 International License (http://creativecommons.org/licenses/by-nc-nd/4.0/), which permits any noncommercial use, sharing, distribution and reproduction in any medium or format, as long as you give appropriate credit to the original author(s) and the source, provide a link to the Creative Commons license and indicate if you modified the licensed material. You do not have permission under this license to share adapted material derived from this chapter or parts of it.

The images or other third party material in this chapter are included in the chapter's Creative Commons license, unless indicated otherwise in a credit line to the material. If material is not included in the chapter's Creative Commons license and your intended use is not permitted by statutory regulation or exceeds the permitted use, you will need to obtain permission directly from the copyright holder.

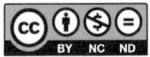

Flowcharts: Approach to Blurring of Vision (Binocular)

Ralene Sim

R. Sim (✉)
Department of Training and Education, Singapore National Eye Centre, Singapore Eye Research Institute, Singapore, Singapore
e-mail: ralene.sim@mohh.com.sg

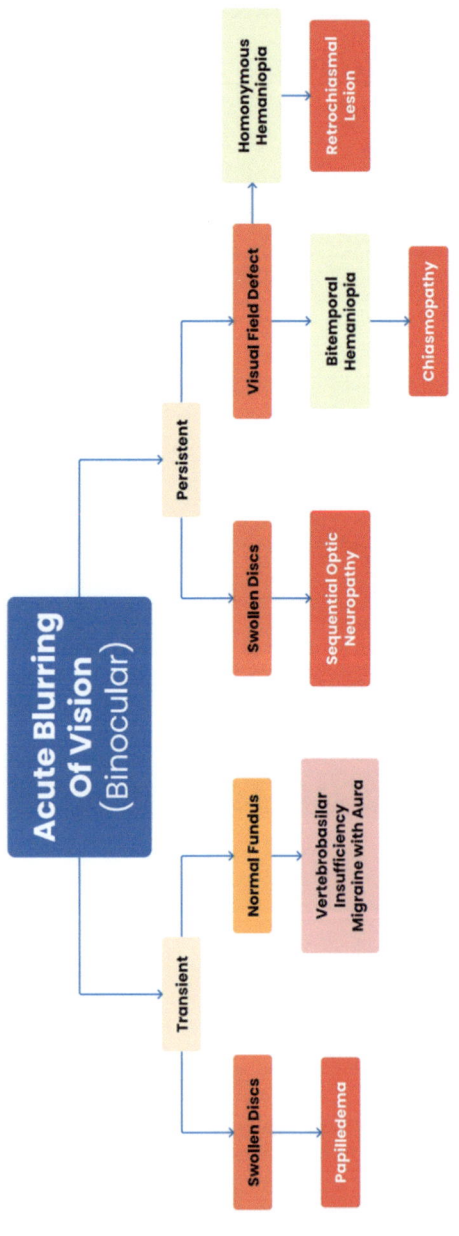

Open Access This chapter is licensed under the terms of the Creative Commons Attribution-NonCommercial-NoDerivatives 4.0 International License (http://creativecommons.org/licenses/by-nc-nd/4.0/), which permits any noncommercial use, sharing, distribution and reproduction in any medium or format, as long as you give appropriate credit to the original author(s) and the source, provide a link to the Creative Commons license and indicate if you modified the licensed material. You do not have permission under this license to share adapted material derived from this chapter or parts of it.

The images or other third party material in this chapter are included in the chapter's Creative Commons license, unless indicated otherwise in a credit line to the material. If material is not included in the chapter's Creative Commons license and your intended use is not permitted by statutory regulation or exceeds the permitted use, you will need to obtain permission directly from the copyright holder.

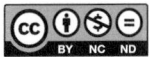

Flowcharts: Approach to Red Eye (Painful)

Ralene Sim

R. Sim (✉)
Department of Training and Education, Singapore National Eye Centre, Singapore Eye Research Institute, Singapore, Singapore
e-mail: ralene.sim@mohh.com.sg

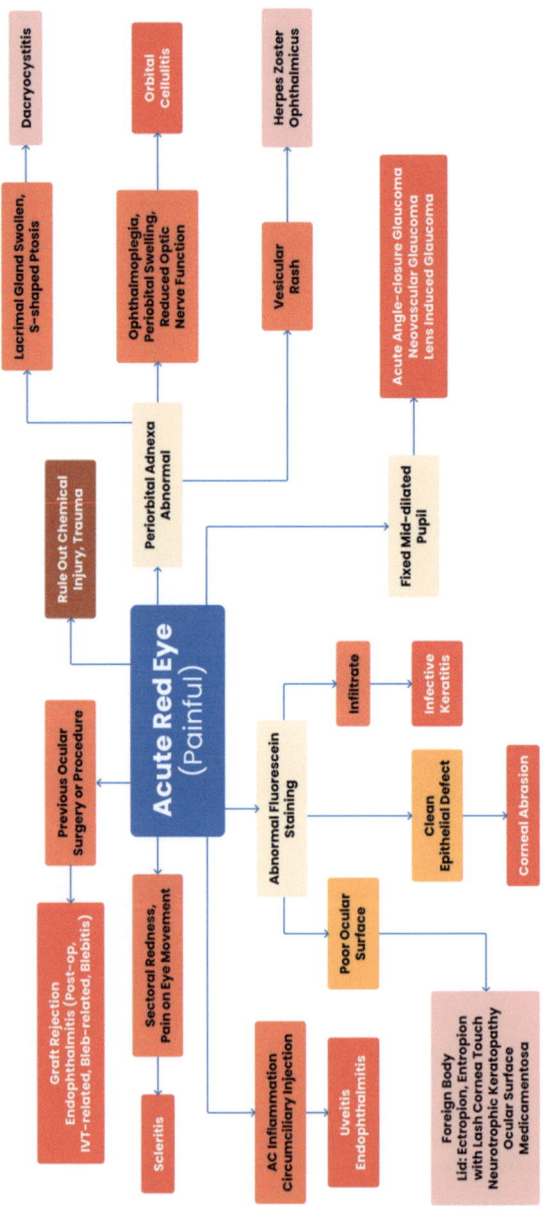

Open Access This chapter is licensed under the terms of the Creative Commons Attribution-NonCommercial-NoDerivatives 4.0 International License (http://creativecommons.org/licenses/by-nc-nd/4.0/), which permits any noncommercial use, sharing, distribution and reproduction in any medium or format, as long as you give appropriate credit to the original author(s) and the source, provide a link to the Creative Commons license and indicate if you modified the licensed material. You do not have permission under this license to share adapted material derived from this chapter or parts of it.

The images or other third party material in this chapter are included in the chapter's Creative Commons license, unless indicated otherwise in a credit line to the material. If material is not included in the chapter's Creative Commons license and your intended use is not permitted by statutory regulation or exceeds the permitted use, you will need to obtain permission directly from the copyright holder.

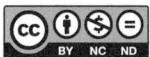

Flowcharts: Approach to Red Eye (Minimal Pain)

4

Ralene Sim

R. Sim (✉)
Department of Training and Education, Singapore National Eye Centre, Singapore Eye Research Institute, Singapore, Singapore
e-mail: ralene.sim@mohh.com.sg

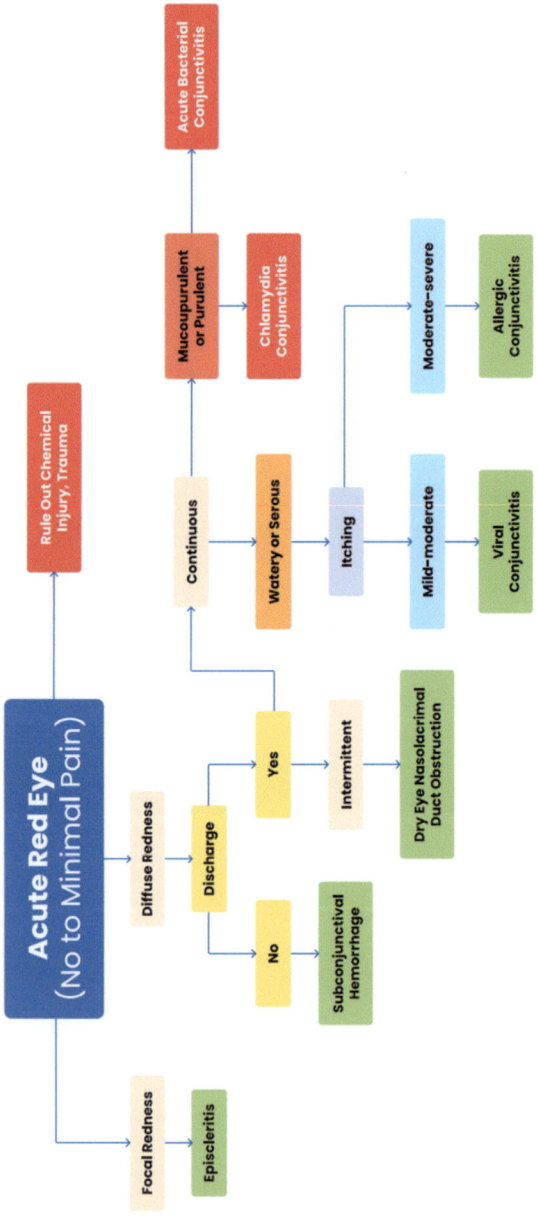

4 Flowcharts: Approach to Red Eye (Minimal Pain)

Open Access This chapter is licensed under the terms of the Creative Commons Attribution-NonCommercial-NoDerivatives 4.0 International License (http://creativecommons.org/licenses/by-nc-nd/4.0/), which permits any noncommercial use, sharing, distribution and reproduction in any medium or format, as long as you give appropriate credit to the original author(s) and the source, provide a link to the Creative Commons license and indicate if you modified the licensed material. You do not have permission under this license to share adapted material derived from this chapter or parts of it.

The images or other third party material in this chapter are included in the chapter's Creative Commons license, unless indicated otherwise in a credit line to the material. If material is not included in the chapter's Creative Commons license and your intended use is not permitted by statutory regulation or exceeds the permitted use, you will need to obtain permission directly from the copyright holder.

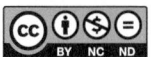

Part II

A Clinical Guide to Ocular Emergencies and Common Ocular Conditions: Ocular Emergencies

Trauma: Corneal Foreign Body

Yap Guan Hui and Melissa Wong

History

- Time and mechanism of injury (e.g. grinding or drilling)
- Nature of foreign body (e.g. metallic, organic material)
- Use of protective eyewear

Examination

- VA
- FB appearance, depth, and location
- Infiltrates or infection
- AC activity
- Evert upper lids ± sweep to exclude retained FBs in fornices
- Fundus exam to exclude intraocular FB (IOFB)

Investigations

- X-ray orbits or CT orbits if IOFB suspected

Y. G. Hui · M. Wong (✉)
Singapore National Eye Centre, Singapore Eye Research Institute,
Singapore, Singapore
e-mail: melissa.wong.h.y@singhealth.com.sg

© The Author(s) 2026
A. C S Tan et al. (eds.), *The Global Eye Health Handbook*,
https://doi.org/10.1007/978-981-96-8861-6_5

Treatment

- Remove corneal FB and rust ring with bent 27-gauge needle under topical anaesthesia. This can be done for visible cornea FB as shown in the following 2 photographs (Figs. 5.1 and 5.2).
- Prophylactic topical antibiotics

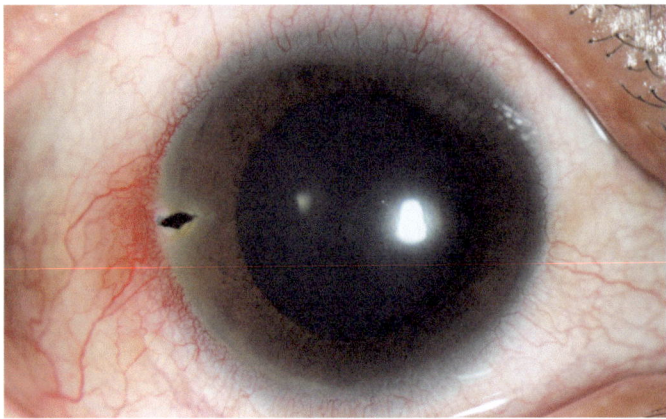

Fig. 5.1 The anterior segment photo of this patient depicts a metallic foreign body in the 9 o'clock region of the peripheral temporal cornea

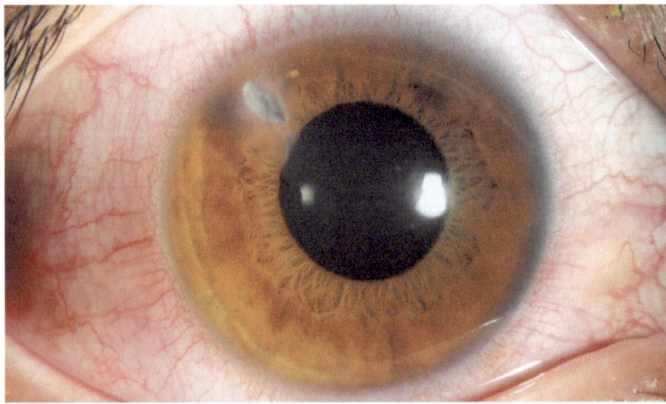

Fig. 5.2 The anterior segment photo of this patient depicts a metallic foreign body in the 11 o'clock region of the superior cornea

- Consider intensive fortified antibiotics for infections
- Follow-up in clinic for removal of residual rust ring and confirmation of epithelial defect closure

Management Tips
- Always ensure sufficient topical anaesthesia and educate the patient on how the corneal scraping will be performed and what the patient must do during scraping to make the process as smooth as possible for both doctor and patient.
- Removal of residual rust rings should be done in a measured fashion. It is preferable to remove the rust ring partially in one sitting and bring the patient back for further removal of the residual rust ring, rather than scraping too deep leaving behind a residual corneal stroma that is too thin.
- If there is an associated infective infiltrate at the site of corneal foreign body, remember to scrape and send for cultures while treating it with broad-spectrum intensive fortified topical antibiotics.
- Take the opportunity during the consultation to educate the patient on protective eyewear to prevent a further episode of corneal or intraocular foreign body injuries.

GEH Perspectives
- *Prioritize Safe Removal*: When removing a corneal foreign body, especially in resource-limited settings, it's crucial to balance the benefits of removing rust rings with the risk of creating corneal scars due to excessive scraping. Aim for gentle, precise removal to minimise scarring and maintain visual clarity. In some cases, leaving a small amount of rust behind and allowing it to resorb naturally may be preferable to causing permanent corneal damage.
- *Sterile Technique*: Always ensure that instruments used for corneal foreign body removal are sterile to avoid introducing infections, particularly in regions where access to follow-up care or antibiotics may be limited.

- *Patient Education and Access to Care*: Educate patients about the signs of infection and the importance of seeking follow-up care if symptoms like increased pain, redness, or vision loss occur. In areas with limited access to healthcare, establishing reliable referral pathways to secondary care centres or using telemedicine can help ensure timely management of post-removal complications

Open Access This chapter is licensed under the terms of the Creative Commons Attribution-NonCommercial-NoDerivatives 4.0 International License (http://creativecommons.org/licenses/by-nc-nd/4.0/), which permits any noncommercial use, sharing, distribution and reproduction in any medium or format, as long as you give appropriate credit to the original author(s) and the source, provide a link to the Creative Commons license and indicate if you modified the licensed material. You do not have permission under this license to share adapted material derived from this chapter or parts of it.

The images or other third party material in this chapter are included in the chapter's Creative Commons license, unless indicated otherwise in a credit line to the material. If material is not included in the chapter's Creative Commons license and your intended use is not permitted by statutory regulation or exceeds the permitted use, you will need to obtain permission directly from the copyright holder.

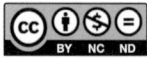

Trauma: Open Globe Injury

Yap Guan Hui and Melissa Wong

History

- Time and mechanism of injury (e.g. grinding or drilling)
- Nature of foreign body (e.g. metallic, organic material)
- Use of protective eyewear
- Medication and treatment history, if any
- Time of last meal/drink

Examination

- AVOID excessive pressure on globe in suspected open globe injuries
- VA and RAPD
- Wound site and size, prolapse of contents, Seidel test
- Anterior segment: Shallow or very deep AC (posterior rupture)
- Traumatic cataract—subluxated/dislocated
- Any breach of anterior/posterior lens capsule to suggest intra-ocular foreign body
- High or low IOP—avoid checking if obvious open globe

- Hypopyon, hyphaemea
- Posterior segment
- IOFB
- Vitreous haemorrhage or vitritis
- Retinal breaks or detachment

Investigations

- X-ray orbits (anterior/posterior in up- and down-gaze, Water's view, lateral)
- CT orbits if suspecting IOFB (usually required)
- Preoperative workup (FBC, Renal panel, CXR, ECG)

Treatment

- Shield the eye
- Admission and keep nil by mouth. Guarded prognosis should be informed in severe open globe injuries as seen in the following photographs (Figs. 6.1 and 6.2).

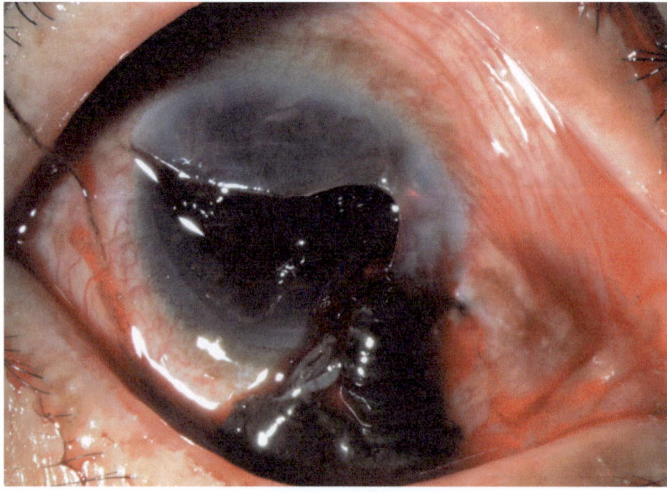

Fig. 6.1 The anterior segment photo shows a ruptured globe with uveal contents prolapsing from the large central corneal laceration

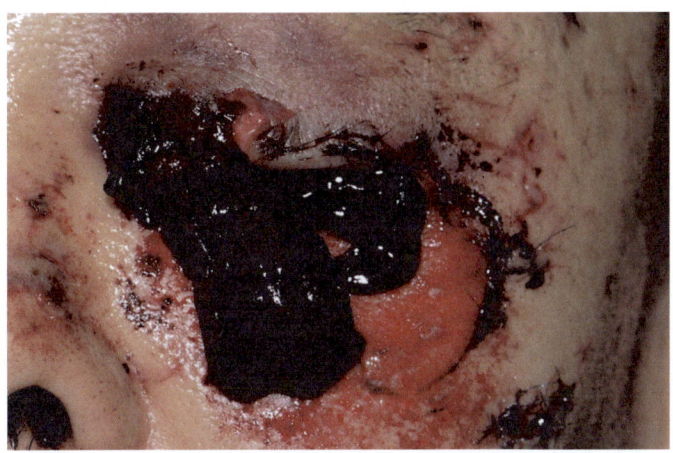

Fig. 6.2 The anterior segment photo shows a disorganised globe that is completely macerated, with the extruded intra-orbital contents obscuring the globe. There is a full-thickness medial upper lid laceration as well

- IM tetanus (check status first)
- Inform registrar/consultant and arrange emergency op
- Primary toilet and suture under non-depolarising general anaesthesia
- Intraoperative swab cultures
- Post-operative antibiotics
- Topical cefazolin and gentamicin hourly
- Oral or intravenous ciprofloxacin
- Close monitoring for infection

Overall Management Principles
- Remember that magnetic resonance imaging is contraindicated in intraocular foreign body injuries, as the foreign body may have metallic magnetic properties, which may dislodge the foreign body and create further trauma to the patient's eye.
- It is important to document the size of the laceration, estimating the extent of it and where the foreign body is, as this can help with surgical planning.

- Non-depolarising general anaesthesia is mandatory to prevent co-contraction of the extraocular muscles, which can lead to increase in intraocular pressure and further extrusion of intraocular contents.
- Usage of Jaffe's speculum or lid traction sutures during draping will help in minimising pressure exerted onto the globe and risks of prolapse of intraocular contents.
- For corneal suturing, to maintain the prolate shape of the cornea. spacing the peripheral corneal sutures more widely apart with longer bites, while placing the corneal sutures closer to each other with shorter bites.

GEH Perspectives

- *Keep Clear Records*: It is always a good idea to document the time of review and any findings carefully. This is especially important in cases of open globe injuries, which can have medico-legal implications. Clear documentation helps ensure accurate follow-up and accountability.
- *Capture the Details*: Whenever possible, take photographs or create simple drawings with rough dimensions of the injury. This can be helpful both for legal reasons and for tracking the healing process over time. Even a quick sketch can make a big difference!
- *Be Prepared for Cultures*: For cases involving severe trauma, having culture plates ready in the operating theatre can be very useful. This ensures that if there's any suspicion of infection, you can take swift action to get the right treatment started.
- *Manage Expectations*: In more severe trauma cases, it is important to keep patients informed about the potential for a guarded prognosis and the possibility of needing multiple surgeries. Setting realistic expectations can help patients and families better cope with the healing process.

Open Access This chapter is licensed under the terms of the Creative Commons Attribution-NonCommercial-NoDerivatives 4.0 International License (http://creativecommons.org/licenses/by-nc-nd/4.0/), which permits any noncommercial use, sharing, distribution and reproduction in any medium or format, as long as you give appropriate credit to the original author(s) and the source, provide a link to the Creative Commons license and indicate if you modified the licensed material. You do not have permission under this license to share adapted material derived from this chapter or parts of it.

The images or other third party material in this chapter are included in the chapter's Creative Commons license, unless indicated otherwise in a credit line to the material. If material is not included in the chapter's Creative Commons license and your intended use is not permitted by statutory regulation or exceeds the permitted use, you will need to obtain permission directly from the copyright holder.

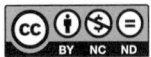

Trauma: Hyphaema

Claire Peterson, Zhu Li Yap, and Sahil Thakur

History

- Blunt orbital trauma and mechanism of injury
- Blurring of vision
- Pain
- History of blood dyscrasias or use of blood-thinners

Examination

- Reduced VA and colour vision, presence of RAPD (reverse method if no view of pupil)
- Raised IOP
- Hyphaema and level (e.g. '8-ball' hyphaema) (Figs. 7.1 and 7.2)
- Corneal blood staining
- Exclude other injuries

C. Peterson · Z. L. Yap (✉) · S. Thakur
Singapore National Eye Centre, Singapore Eye Research Institute, Singapore, Singapore
e-mail: yap.zhu.li@singhealth.com.sg

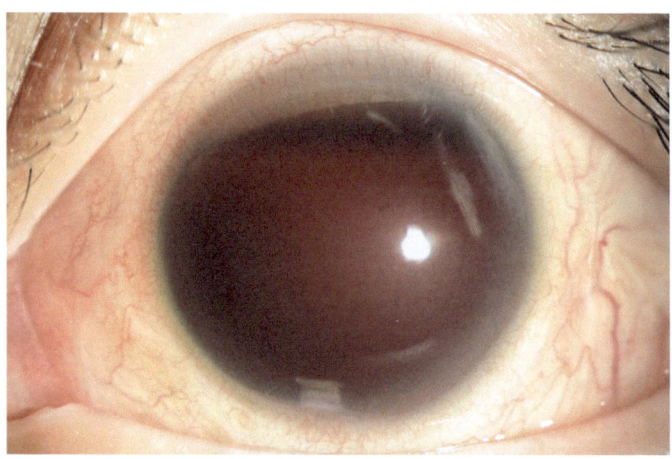

Fig. 7.1 The anterior segment photo shows a near-total hyphaema occluding the entire visual axis, with corneal blood staining superiorly

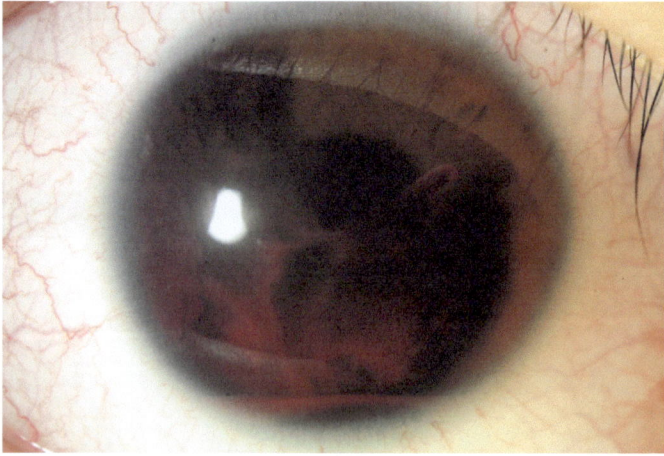

Fig. 7.2 The anterior segment photograph shows a gross hyphaema obscuring the visual axis that is slowly consolidating in layers with the superior pupil edge just visible

Investigations

- Ultrasound B-scan if posterior segment not visualised

Treatment

- Consider admission in these cases
  - Paediatric patients
  - High IOP
  - 8-ball hyphaema
- Bed rest and limited physical activity
- Cycloplegics
- Topical steroids
- Glaucoma medications
- Surgical washout for persistent high IOP and non-resolving hyphaema (risk of corneal staining or glaucomatous optic neuropathy)

> **GEH Perspectives**
> - *Review Medications*: If safe to do so, consider stopping anticoagulants and NSAIDs to reduce the risk of further bleeding, but always consult with the medical team to weigh the risks and benefits.
> - *Stay Alert for Re-bleeds*: Be especially vigilant for re-bleeding within the first 5–7 days, as this is a critical period for recurrence.
> - *Think Ahead for Children*: In pediatric cases at risk of amblyopia, consider early anterior chamber (AC) washout to prevent long-term visual impairment.
> - *Prevent IOP Spikes*: Anticipate a rise in intraocular pressure (IOP) and consider using glaucoma medications prophylactically to protect the optic nerve.

Open Access This chapter is licensed under the terms of the Creative Commons Attribution-NonCommercial-NoDerivatives 4.0 International License (http://creativecommons.org/licenses/by-nc-nd/4.0/), which permits any noncommercial use, sharing, distribution and reproduction in any medium or format, as long as you give appropriate credit to the original author(s) and the source, provide a link to the Creative Commons license and indicate if you modified the licensed material. You do not have permission under this license to share adapted material derived from this chapter or parts of it.

The images or other third party material in this chapter are included in the chapter's Creative Commons license, unless indicated otherwise in a credit line to the material. If material is not included in the chapter's Creative Commons license and your intended use is not permitted by statutory regulation or exceeds the permitted use, you will need to obtain permission directly from the copyright holder.

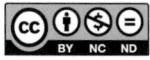

Trauma: Orbital Fracture

8

Yap Guan Hui and Yvonne Chung

History

- Time and mechanism of injury
- Blurring of vision
- Ocular pain especially with movement
- Diplopia
- Presence of nausea and light-headedness especially in particular directions of gaze
- Take note particularly if workplace injury or assault (may have criminal or legal ramifications)

Examination

- Proptosis or enophthalmos
- Periorbital swelling and bruising
- Eyelid/skin injuries, e.g. lacerations
- Check optic nerve function: visual acuity, colour vision, visual fields, RAPD

Y. G. Hui · Y. Chung (✉)
Singapore National Eye Centre, Singapore Eye Research Institute, Singapore, Singapore
e-mail: chung.hsi.wei@singhealth.com.sg

- Limitation of extraocular motility (remove especially on upgaze—depends where the fracture is located), pain on eye movements, presence of oculocardiac reflex
- Orbital rim step deformities, periorbital crepitus
- Infraorbital hypoaesthesia
- If ptosis is present, check levator palpebrae superioris function
- Complete ocular examination as per assessment for open globe injury (can remove all the ocular examination points)

Anterior Segment

- Traumatic hyphaema and mydriasis
- Iridodialysis
- Phacodonesis

Posterior Segment

- Vitreous haemorrhage
- Retinal breaks and detachment
- Commotio retinae

Investigations

- Orbital X-rays as a minimum for all medicolegal cases
- Maxillary haemoantrum, teardrop sign (herniation of orbital contents through the orbital floor)
- Consider CT orbits if significant limitation of extraocular motility/enophthalmos (especially if entrapment is suspected), infraorbital hypoaesthesia present or significant fracture seen on X-ray orbits
- Hess chart and binocular single vision (BSV) and facial photographs with nine directions of gaze if significant diplopia, planned for fracture repair or in potential legal/criminal cases

Treatment

- Urgent CT orbits keep in view admission and urgent surgery in cases of extraocular muscle entrapment (mainly children)
- Conservative non-surgical management is appropriate in situations such as:
  - Elderly, who is not fit or keen for surgery
  - No extraocular motility restriction/diplopia, minimally displaced fractures, asymptomatic
  - Conservative management: Oral Co-amoxiclav 1 g BD for 1 week, advise not to blow nose, cold compresses to reduce bruising and swelling
- Surgical repair is indicated for
  - Large, displaced fractures
  - Symptomatic with pain on extraocular motility/diplopia/enophthalmos
- A HESS/BSV test can be requested preoperatively for documentation

Clinical Pearls

- Always document the presence of diplopia, extraocular muscle (EOM) limitation, and infraorbital hypoesthesia—these findings may change post-operatively if patient undergoes repair
- Beware of young patients with a white eye and EOM limitation with associated nausea and feeling unwell/bradycardia—potential greenstick fracture with entrapment of extraocular muscles requiring urgent surgery ("white eye blowout fracture")
- Medicolegal cases: assault, suspected domestic violence, suspected child abuse, worksite or school injuries, road traffic accidents, prison, persons under custody, military duty, unconscious

GEH Perspectives

- *Assessing the Fracture*: If your patient is not experiencing diplopia, significant globe dystopia, or enophthalmos, it may be reasonable to monitor them clinically after the initial swelling goes down. This approach can be particularly useful in areas where radiological imaging is limited.
- *Basic Imaging First*: An orbital or facial X-ray is often sufficient for screening when there are no major signs or symptoms of an orbital wall fracture. If concerns persist, you can always consider more detailed imaging, like a computed tomography (CT) scan, later on if surgical repair may be necessary.
- *Surgical Repair Not Always Needed*: Just because a fracture is present doesn't mean surgery is required right away. If there is no muscle entrapment and the swelling from the injury has resolved, orbital fractures without ongoing diplopia or significant enophthalmos can often be managed conservatively.

Open Access This chapter is licensed under the terms of the Creative Commons Attribution-NonCommercial-NoDerivatives 4.0 International License (http://creativecommons.org/licenses/by-nc-nd/4.0/), which permits any non-commercial use, sharing, distribution and reproduction in any medium or format, as long as you give appropriate credit to the original author(s) and the source, provide a link to the Creative Commons license and indicate if you modified the licensed material. You do not have permission under this license to share adapted material derived from this chapter or parts of it.

The images or other third party material in this chapter are included in the chapter's Creative Commons license, unless indicated otherwise in a credit line to the material. If material is not included in the chapter's Creative Commons license and your intended use is not permitted by statutory regulation or exceeds the permitted use, you will need to obtain permission directly from the copyright holder.

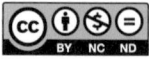

Trauma: Eyelid Lacerations

Yap Guan Hui and Yvonne Chung

History

- Mechanism of injury, e.g. blunt force causing avulsion or sharp injury causing laceration, dog bite, risk of foreign body
- Time and context of injury—potential legal/criminal case?
- Associated ocular symptoms e.g. blurring of vision, diplopia to assess for concomitant ocular/orbital injuries such as open globe, orbital fractures

Examination

- Exclude sight-threatening injuries first e.g. open globe injury—refer to appropriate chapter.
- Exclude orbital fractures—refer to appropriate chapter.
- Assess eyelid wound—document location, extent, and depth.
- Involving lid margin?
- Medial to punctum/lateral displacement of punctum? (risk of canalicular injury)—will need careful probing and syringing to assess patency of canalicular system

Y. G. Hui · Y. Chung (✉)
Singapore National Eye Centre, Singapore Eye Research Institute, Singapore, Singapore
e-mail: chung.hsi.wei@singhealth.com.sg

- Presence of tissue loss?
- Presence of orbital fat (high risk of underlying open globe injury)—examine eye very carefully especially underneath location of lid injury, particularly if subconjunctival haemorrhage is also present—may mask globe rupture/laceration wound.
- Presence of ptosis? Document lid measurements including levator palpebrae superioris function.
- Assess eyes for any concomitant ocular trauma sustained.

Investigations

- Consider urgent CT orbits if there is suspicion of penetrating injury, severe blunt trauma, or intraocular/intraorbital foreign bodies

Treatment

- Intramuscular Tetanus injection immediately.
- Copious wound irrigation and removal of visible foreign particles in wound.
- Consider oral antibiotics, e.g. oral augmentin 1 g twice a day for a week if dirty wound or high risk of infection.
- If sparing eyelid margin, for primary closure with 6-0 or 7-0 silk or nylon to skin, topical antibiotics to skin wound e.g. tobramycin ointment three times a day or Fucithalmic ointment twice a day, follow up in 5–7 days for removal of sutures.
- If involving eyelid margin/canalicular system/significant tissue loss/visible orbital fat prolapse/presence of intraorbital foreign body, refer to the oculoplastics team.
- If simple eyelid margin-involving laceration, e.g. canalicular system is not involved, no significant tissue loss is present, and there is no orbital fat prolapse, consider primary closure with:
    - 6-0 silk to appose grey line and lash line (taking care to avoid lid notching and leaving suture ends long for incorporation to skin sutures subsequently).

- 6-0 Vicryl to appose tarsus.
- 6-0 or 7-0 silk or nylon to skin with incorporation of grey line and lash line sutures.
- Topical antibiotics to wound.
- Refer to oculoplastics team on call for follow-up plans, consider removal of sutures in 7–10 days.

Clinical Pearls

- Carefully document wound features with diagrams or photographs if possible.
- Keep patient fasted while referring to the oculoplastics team in cases of canalicular involvement as urgent repair within 24–48 h will be required.
- Be highly suspicious of tissue loss in dog bite or gouging mechanisms of injury.
- Be highly suspicious of underlying open globe injuries if orbital fat prolapse is present, i.e. the orbital septum has been breached (Fig. 9.1).
- Counsel patients about risks of lid margin notching and lagophthalmos post-repair if lid margin is involved.

GEH Perspectives
- *Prevent Complications*: It is crucial to prioritise tetanus injections, clean the wound properly, and consider antibiotic therapy to prevent any secondary infections. These steps help ensure a smoother recovery for your patients.
- *Educate Your Patients*: Make sure patients fully understand their injuries and the proposed treatment options. It is important for them to be aware of the potential consequences of conservative management. For instance, in resource-limited settings where access to an operating theatre might be restricted, let them know that not repairing canalicular lacerations can lead to ongoing tearing and permanent disfigurement. Clear communication helps them make informed decisions about their care.

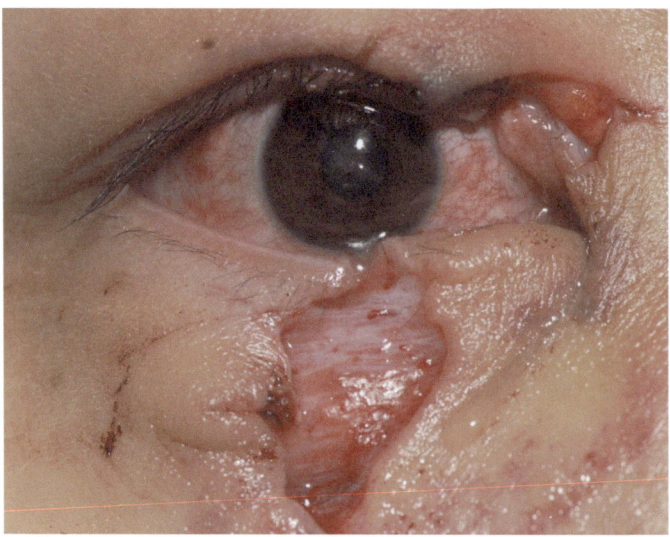

Fig. 9.1 The above half-face photo shows an upper and lower margin-involving lid laceration with septum breach and exposure of the underlying orbicularis muscle. There is also another lid laceration involving the medial canthal area which is suspicious for canalicular involvement

Open Access This chapter is licensed under the terms of the Creative Commons Attribution-NonCommercial-NoDerivatives 4.0 International License (http://creativecommons.org/licenses/by-nc-nd/4.0/), which permits any noncommercial use, sharing, distribution and reproduction in any medium or format, as long as you give appropriate credit to the original author(s) and the source, provide a link to the Creative Commons license and indicate if you modified the licensed material. You do not have permission under this license to share adapted material derived from this chapter or parts of it.

The images or other third party material in this chapter are included in the chapter's Creative Commons license, unless indicated otherwise in a credit line to the material. If material is not included in the chapter's Creative Commons license and your intended use is not permitted by statutory regulation or exceeds the permitted use, you will need to obtain permission directly from the copyright holder.

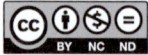

Trauma: Traumatic Optic Neuropathy (TON)

Reuben Foo, Shweta Singhal, and Umapathi Thirugnanam

History

- High-velocity closed-head trauma
- Loss of consciousness
- Blurring of vision

Examination

- Reduced visual acuity (VA) and colour vision, presence of relative afferent pupillary defect (RAPD)
- Visual field defects

Investigations

- Orbital CT with fine (1 mm) cuts, specifying focus on any fragments in optic canal.
- Look for bone fragments and optic nerve compression along the optic canal.
- If none is seen, could be indirect optic nerve trauma.

R. Foo · S. Singhal (✉) · U. Thirugnanam
Singapore National Eye Centre, Singapore Eye Research Institute, Singapore, Singapore
e-mail: shweta.singhal@singhealth.com.sg

Treatment

- Inform Oculoplastics and neuro-ophthalmology teams.
- Surgical priority for intracranial bleeds/unstable facial fracture treatment.
- If there is clear bony impingement of optic nerve, surgical treatment of TON may be considered but itself carries a risk of blindness. Procedure should only be done if the patient is alert enough to understand risks of the procedure.
- No evidence for benefit with systemic steroid therapy (high or low dose)—the latter has fewer side effects so can be offered empirically (intravenous (IV) Methylprednisolone 1 g/day × 3 days) in cases with very poor vision.
- 50% of cases show some spontaneous recovery.
- Warn of guarded visual prognosis.

> **GEH Perspectives**
> - *Understanding Treatment Limitations*: It is important to note that there isn't an effective treatment for TON. However, be aware that about 50% of cases can show spontaneous improvement, although the extent of this improvement can vary.
> - *Surgical Considerations*: Surgical decompression of bony impingement should only be considered if the patient is alert enough to understand the risks of the procedure. Ensure that they are informed and engaged in the decision-making process.
> - *Steroid Therapy*: High-dose steroid therapy is not recommended for TON, so it's best to avoid offering this option. However, low-dose steroid therapy can be provided on an empirical basis if deemed appropriate.

Open Access This chapter is licensed under the terms of the Creative Commons Attribution-NonCommercial-NoDerivatives 4.0 International License (http://creativecommons.org/licenses/by-nc-nd/4.0/), which permits any noncommercial use, sharing, distribution and reproduction in any medium or format, as long as you give appropriate credit to the original author(s) and the source, provide a link to the Creative Commons license and indicate if you modified the licensed material. You do not have permission under this license to share adapted material derived from this chapter or parts of it.

The images or other third party material in this chapter are included in the chapter's Creative Commons license, unless indicated otherwise in a credit line to the material. If material is not included in the chapter's Creative Commons license and your intended use is not permitted by statutory regulation or exceeds the permitted use, you will need to obtain permission directly from the copyright holder.

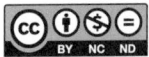

Infections: Infective Keratitis

Nicole Sie, Marcus Ang, and Anshu Arundhati

Introduction to Cornea

Corneal disease is a major cause of visual impairment and blindness worldwide, particularly in low- and middle-income countries. Unlike other causes of blindness such as cataract or glaucoma, corneal blindness is often preventable and affects individuals across all age groups, including young adults and children. Causes vary geographically but commonly include infections and trauma, including chemical injury. Managing corneal disease requires early recognition, prompt treatment, and, in some cases, access to advanced surgical care—resources that may not always be available in under-resourced settings. Community-based approaches focusing on prevention, early detection, and appropriate referral are essential to reduce the burden of corneal blindness.

N. Sie · A. Arundhati
Singapore National Eye Centre, Singapore Eye Research Institute, Singapore, Singapore

M. Ang (✉)
Department of Cornea and External Eye, Singapore National Eye Centre, Singapore Eye Research Institute, Singapore, Singapore
e-mail: marcus.Ang@Singhealth.com.sg

© The Author(s) 2026
A. C S Tan et al. (eds.), *The Global Eye Health Handbook*,
https://doi.org/10.1007/978-981-96-8861-6_11

Prompt Identification and Early Management

Cornea pathology can be acute and sight-threatening if not detected early and promptly managed. It is crucial that general ophthalmologists and allied health staff are able to identify and triage these cases accordingly when they present to emergency settings and to dispense initial management to the best of their abilities in settings where resources may be limited. It is crucial to then have in place a set of standardised referral pathways where prompt referral can be made to corneal surgeons if local general ophthalmologists are unable to further manage these cases.

Reliable Documentation and Slit Lamp Photography

Maintaining comprehensive records for each patient, including relevant slit lamp photographs or detailed corneal sketches (if slit lamp photography is unavailable), is essential for managing corneal pathology effectively. Such documentation ensures continuity of care, especially when patients may not have access to follow-up with the same physician.

In cases of infectious keratitis, it is beneficial for regions or countries to establish an infectious keratitis registry to monitor local pathogens and resistance patterns. Tracking these trends can guide the selection of first-line broad-spectrum agents, supporting more effective and targeted treatment of bacterial infections.

Patient Education

- It is equally important to educate our patients on the importance of eye health and common acute eye conditions which require them to seek prompt medical attention without delay. Patient education initiatives such as advertisements in local media or through leaflets or flyers or even online educational seminars carried out by healthcare professionals should be used to distribute knowledge to local populations in their native dialect.

History

- Risk factors for infection
  - Contact lens (CL) history (type, duration, cleaning, hygiene, previous infections)
  - Trauma (foreign body, corneal abrasion)
  - Underlying ocular disease (e.g. neurotrophic cornea, exposure/lagophthalmos/eyelid malposition/abnormal eyelashes, recurrent corneal erosions)
  - Contact with soil or vegetative matter or water (e.g. showers/hot tubs/swimming pools)
  - Previous ocular surgery
  - Long-term steroid eye drops use
- Symptoms and duration
  - Pain
  - Blurring of vision
  - Redness
  - Photophobia
- Prior treatment (e.g. topical antibiotics or steroids)

Examination

- Eyelids and adnexa
  - Eyelid malpositions/abnormal eyelashes
  - Lagophthalmos
  - Blepharitis or meibomian gland disease
  - Evert eyelids to exclude subtotal conjunctival foreign bodies
- Conjunctival injection
- Corneal ulcer description
  - Location, depth, dimensions
  - Overlying extent of epithelial defect
  - Associated thinning
  - Appearance of edges (e.g. ground glass, feathery)
  - Radial perineuritis
  - Satellite lesions
- Anterior chamber cells, flare, hypopyon, and fibrin
- Dilated fundus examination TRO endophthalmitis (Fig. 11.1).

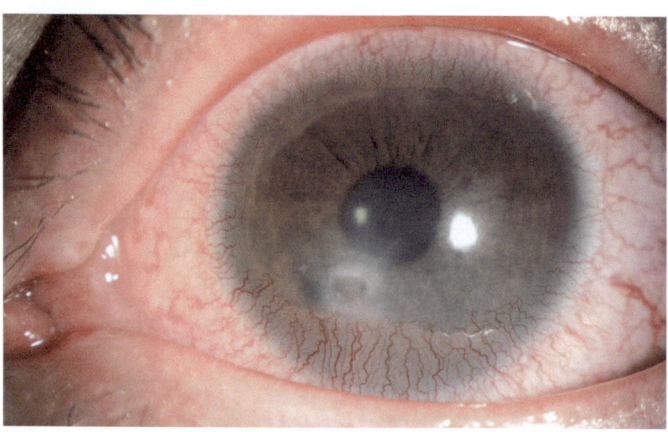

Fig. 11.1 Contact lens-related keratitis. This anterior segment photo of the left eye depicts an active inferonasal corneal infiltrate with peripheral vascularisation and pannus from chronic contact lens overuse

Investigations

- Corneal slit lamp photographs if available, or drawings to document
- Corneal scrapings (send CL, casing, and cleaning solution if available)
- (1) Slide for Gram stain (± KOH if suspicious for fungus)
- Culture media: (2) blood agar, (3) chocolate agar, (4) brain heart infusion broth (BHIB), (5) thioglycolate broth, (6) Sabouraud agar (± non-nutrient agar with *E. coli* overlay for suspected *Acanthamoeba*—requires 1 h preparation during office hours)
- Consider conjunctival swab for cases with severe thinning

How to Perform a Corneal Scraping

- Instil preservative free topical anaesthetic eye drops
- Use a new (bent) 27G needle or Kimura spatula

- Change needles or sterilise Kimura spatula between each scrape
- Remove overlying discharge or slough
- Scrape at the active edge of the ulcer to improve diagnostic yield
- Ulcer material should be clearly visible on the needle for each scrape
- Instruct patient to keep forehead pressing against the strap to reduce risk of inadvertent perforation

Treatment

- Remove causative agent if present, e.g.
  - Epilate abnormal lashes
  - Treat underlying exposure or eyelid malpositions, if present
  - Stop steroid eye drops
- Fortified preservative free cefazolin (50 mg/mL) and gentamicin (14 mg/mL) hourly throughout the day and night
- Cycloplegia (e.g. homatropine or atropine) for photophobia
- +/− Oral analgesia for severe pain
- Oral ciprofloxacin 500 mg twice daily for lesions that
  - Extend to the limbus
  - Have severe thinning or impending corneal perforation
  - Large ulcers
  - Ulcers in close proximity to intraocular wounds
  - Associated hypopyon
- Avoid use of topical medications in cases of perforation
- Consider admission in certain cases (e.g. large ulcer, central or paracentral location, patient unable to manage frequent eye drops or return for frequent follow-up)
- Trace cornea cultures and sensitivities and tailor antibiotic regimen accordingly
- Severe cases with limited response to treatment or those resulting in perforation may need surgical therapeutic or tectonic keratoplasty

> **GEH Perspectives**
> - *Consider Risks of Trauma*: Always assess the risk of trauma, especially if there's a high likelihood of vegetative contamination. Fungal infections can be significant sources of keratitis, so it's wise to have a low threshold for starting antifungal treatment when you suspect this type of contamination
> - *Use Broad-Spectrum Antibiotics*: Since multiple microbes can be at play in infective keratitis, starting broad-spectrum antibiotic therapy is a good approach. Make sure to cover both Gram-negative and Gram-positive bacteria until you receive definitive histological or culture results. This helps ensure that you're addressing all potential infections effectively.
> - *Be Mindful of Resistance*: With rising global resistance to levofloxacin, it may be time to reconsider traditional antibiotics as first-line options. Staying informed about local resistance patterns can help you choose the most effective treatment for your patients.

Open Access This chapter is licensed under the terms of the Creative Commons Attribution-NonCommercial-NoDerivatives 4.0 International License (http://creativecommons.org/licenses/by-nc-nd/4.0/), which permits any noncommercial use, sharing, distribution and reproduction in any medium or format, as long as you give appropriate credit to the original author(s) and the source, provide a link to the Creative Commons license and indicate if you modified the licensed material. You do not have permission under this license to share adapted material derived from this chapter or parts of it.

The images or other third party material in this chapter are included in the chapter's Creative Commons license, unless indicated otherwise in a credit line to the material. If material is not included in the chapter's Creative Commons license and your intended use is not permitted by statutory regulation or exceeds the permitted use, you will need to obtain permission directly from the copyright holder.

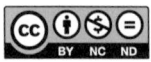

Infections: Conjunctivitis

Nicole Sie, Marcus Ang, and Anshu Arundhati

Common differentials: Adenoviral/Bacterial/Neonatal.

History

Viral Conjunctivitis
- Recent contact with conjunctivitis case(s)
- Recent upper respiratory tract infection
- Acute onset of redness, swelling, tearing, itch, and discomfort
- Typically starts in one eye and spreads to the other eye

Bacterial Conjunctivitis
- Rapid onset
- Purulent or hyper-purulent discharge
- Pain
- Blurring of vision
- History of sexually transmitted infections or high-risk sexual activity

N. Sie · A. Arundhati
Singapore National Eye Centre, Singapore Eye Research Institute, Singapore, Singapore

M. Ang (✉)
Department of Cornea and External Eye, Singapore National Eye Centre, Singapore Eye Research Institute, Singapore, Singapore
e-mail: marcus.Ang@Singhealth.com.sg

© The Author(s) 2026
A. C S Tan et al. (eds.), *The Global Eye Health Handbook*,
https://doi.org/10.1007/978-981-96-8861-6_12

Neonatal Conjunctivitis
- Eye redness and discharge in 1st month of life (usually first 2 weeks)

Examination

Viral Conjunctivitis
- Conjunctival injection, chemosis, subconjunctival haemorrhage
- Follicles over tarsal conjunctiva
- Pseudomembranes over tarsal conjunctiva
- Secondary ocular surface pathology
  - PEEs and filaments and epithelial defects (usually in pseudomembranous)
  - Subepithelial infiltrates
- Enlarged/tender preauricular lymph nodes

Bacterial Conjunctivitis
- Purulent/hyper-purulent discharge
- Gonococcal conjunctivitis usually presents with hyper-purulent discharge
- Conjunctival injection and chemosis
- Secondary cornea ED/melt/perforation

Neonatal Conjunctivitis
- Conjunctival injection and discharge
- Secondary corneal ED (Figs. 12.1 and 12.2)

12 Infections: Conjunctivitis

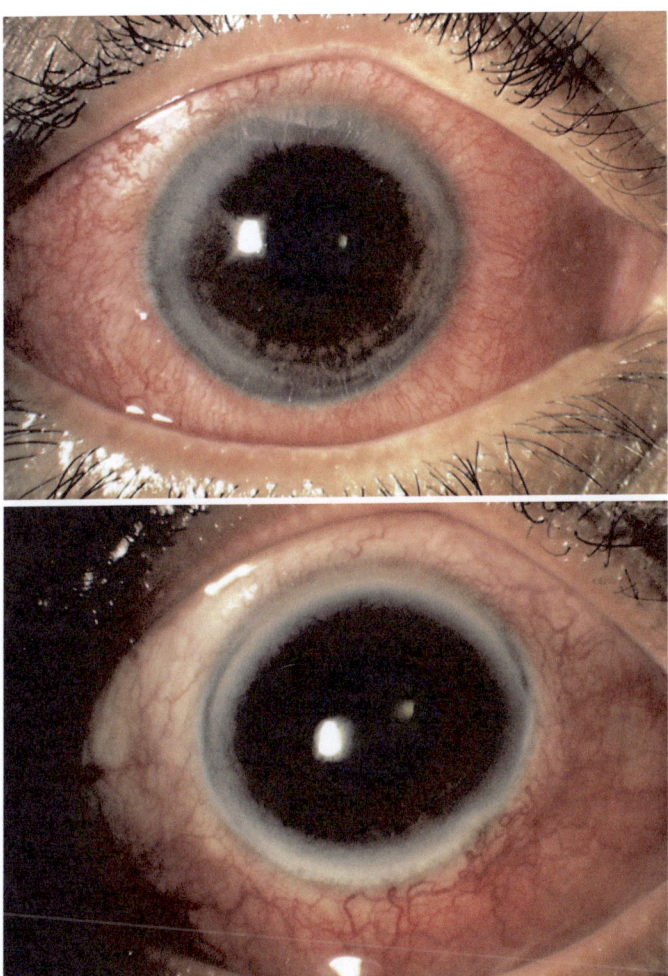

Figs. 12.1 and 12.2 The anterior segment photos above show bilateral diffuse conjunctival injection in a patient with bilateral conjunctivitis. On eversion of the lids, there is presence of diffuse follicles

Investigations

Adenoviral Conjunctivitis
- No investigations needed

Bacterial Conjunctivitis
- Conjunctival swab for Gram stain and cultures
- Gram stain: Gram negative diplococci (*Neisseria gonorrhoeae*)
- Giemsa stain: Basophilic intracytoplasmic inclusion bodies (Chlamydia)
- Chlamydia PCR and immunofluorescence
- Urine culture and cultures

Neonatal Conjunctivitis
- Conjunctival swab for Gram stain and cultures (as listed above under bacterial conjunctivitis)
- Chlamydia PCR and immunofluorescence

Treatment

- Viral Conjunctivitis
  - Remove pseudomembranes
  - Frequent use of preservative-free lubricants
  - Consider topical antibiotics and steroids in case of cornea involvement or pseudomembranes formation
  - Advise patients on importance of hand hygiene and risk of transmission
- *If gonococcal/neonatal conjunctivitis is suspected*:
  - Tetracyclines
  - Referral to an infectious disease and/or neonatology for systemic screening and management
  - Oral azithromycin twice a day for 3 days or IM/IV ceftriaxone
- Supportive treatment in all cases: lid and ocular surface hygiene, aggressive topical preservative-free lubrication, antibiotics for secondary infections, and cold compresses

Trachoma

- Risk Factors:
  - Endemic geographical regions (parts of North Africa, Middle East, North West India, parts of Southeast Asia)
  - Limited environmental and social hygiene resources
  - Poor facial hygiene
  - Overcrowded living conditions

Clinical Features of Trachoma
- Active Disease
  - Follicular conjunctivitis or papillary hypertrophy
  - Corneal pannus
- Potential Serious Complications:
  - Conjunctival scarring
  - Cicatricial entropion and trichiasis
  - Corneal scarring and vascularisation
  - (Herbert's pits: large scarred limbal follicles)

GEH Perspectives
- *Hand Hygiene Is Key*: Always practice and emphasise strict hand hygiene in all cases of conjunctivitis! This simple step can significantly reduce the spread of infection and help protect both patients and healthcare providers.
- *Be Cautious with Pseudomembranes*: If pseudomembranes are present, let your patients know that they may bleed upon removal. This way, they can be prepared for the possibility and understand that it is part of the process.
- *Monitor for Infiltrates*: Keep in mind that subepithelial infiltrates may develop about 2 weeks after the onset of adenoviral keratoconjunctivitis. Educating your patients about this timeline can help them manage their expectations.
- *Support with Medical Leave*: When necessary, provide adequate medical leave for patients. This allows them the time they need to recover fully and helps prevent the spread of conjunctivitis in their communities.

Open Access This chapter is licensed under the terms of the Creative Commons Attribution-NonCommercial-NoDerivatives 4.0 International License (http://creativecommons.org/licenses/by-nc-nd/4.0/), which permits any noncommercial use, sharing, distribution and reproduction in any medium or format, as long as you give appropriate credit to the original author(s) and the source, provide a link to the Creative Commons license and indicate if you modified the licensed material. You do not have permission under this license to share adapted material derived from this chapter or parts of it.

The images or other third party material in this chapter are included in the chapter's Creative Commons license, unless indicated otherwise in a credit line to the material. If material is not included in the chapter's Creative Commons license and your intended use is not permitted by statutory regulation or exceeds the permitted use, you will need to obtain permission directly from the copyright holder.

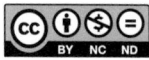

Infections: Onchocerciasis

Nicole Sie, Marcus Ang, and Anshu Arundhati

History

- Ocular symptoms (can be several years later after dermatologic): insidious onset of decreased vision, eye redness, eye pain, and photophobia—often manifest in the fourth to fifth decade
- Dermatologic symptoms: severe pruritus
- Other systemic symptoms: CNS, urinary system

Examination Ocular Exam

- Eyelid—eyelid nodules and oedema
- Conjunctiva—chronic conjunctivitis, chemosis, phlyctenule-like kerato-conjunctival lesions; direct invasion of microfilariae into cornea and sclera
- Cornea—sclerosing keratitis.
- Anterior chamber—iridocyclitis

N. Sie · A. Arundhati
Singapore National Eye Centre, Singapore Eye Research Institute, Singapore, Singapore

M. Ang (✉)
Department of Cornea and External Eye, Singapore National Eye Centre, Singapore Eye Research Institute, Singapore, Singapore
e-mail: marcus.Ang@Singhealth.com.sg

- Corectopia, iris atrophy, cataract
- IOP: Secondary glaucoma from extensive synechiae
- Direct visualisation of microfilaria in anterior chamber or cornea—Nematodes can be seen using retro-illumination as S- or C-shaped fine motile elements—To mobilise the microfilariae that are suspended in anterior chamber, patients can be asked to sit with their head between their knees for at least 2 min
- Fundus exam: chorioretinal lesions, peripapillary chorioretinitis, optic nerve dysfunction secondary to optic nerve oedema and optic neuritis, eventually leading to optic atrophy

Systemic exam Full dermatologic exam: freely mobile subcutaneous nodules measuring 0.5–3 cm in diameter over bony prominences (especially over hips and lower limbs), dermatitis

Investigations

- Clinical confirmation: superficial bloodless skin snip biopsies

Management

- Co-manage with infectious disease specialist
- Standard treatment: broad-spectrum antiparasitic ivermectin, given as a single dose and repeated every 6–12 months over a course of around 10 years
- Symptomatic treatment for acute complications: topical steroids and cycloplegic medications for iridocyclitis

> **GEH Perspectives**
> - *Understand the Impact*: Remember that onchocerciasis is the second leading cause of infectious blindness worldwide and can affect all ocular tissues. Raising awareness about this disease is crucial for prevention and early detection.

- *Promote Individual Prevention*: Encourage individuals in endemic areas to take protective measures against black fly bites. This can include avoiding known hotspots for the disease, using insect repellent, and wearing protective clothing to minimise exposure.
- *Emphasis on Early Detection and Treatment*: Stress that the prognosis of onchocerciasis greatly depends on how early the infection is detected and treated. If treated early, patients can avoid serious complications, while late treatment may lead to irreversible blindness. Educating patients about the importance of seeking medical help promptly can significantly improve their outcomes.

Open Access This chapter is licensed under the terms of the Creative Commons Attribution-NonCommercial-NoDerivatives 4.0 International License (http://creativecommons.org/licenses/by-nc-nd/4.0/), which permits any non-commercial use, sharing, distribution and reproduction in any medium or format, as long as you give appropriate credit to the original author(s) and the source, provide a link to the Creative Commons license and indicate if you modified the licensed material. You do not have permission under this license to share adapted material derived from this chapter or parts of it.

The images or other third party material in this chapter are included in the chapter's Creative Commons license, unless indicated otherwise in a credit line to the material. If material is not included in the chapter's Creative Commons license and your intended use is not permitted by statutory regulation or exceeds the permitted use, you will need to obtain permission directly from the copyright holder.

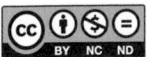

Infections: Herpes Zoster Ophthalmicus (HZO)

Nicole Sie, Marcus Ang, and Anshu Arundhati

History

- Acute onset of erythematous papules/vesicles
- History of chickenpox infection, immunosuppression
- Symptoms:
  - BOV, redness, tearing, photophobia
  - Periorbital swelling and erythema
  - Neuropathic pain over distribution of CNV_1
  - Diplopia

Examination

- Erythematous vesicular rash over the CNV_1 dermatome
- Vesicles along tip of nose (Hutchinson sign)
- Reduced VA +/− RAPD and other signs of optic neuropathy
- Raised IOP (in herpetic uveitis)
- Ptosis and EOM limitation (cranial nerve palsies are common)

N. Sie · A. Arundhati
Singapore National Eye Centre, Singapore Eye Research Institute, Singapore, Singapore

M. Ang (✉)
Department of Cornea and External Eye, Singapore National Eye Centre, Singapore Eye Research Institute, Singapore, Singapore
e-mail: marcus.Ang@Singhealth.com.sg

- Slit lamp examination
  - Conjunctival hyperaemia
  - Corneal hypoesthesia with PEEs and pseudo-dendritic lesions
  - AC cells, flare, posterior synechiae and raised IOP
  - Vitritis, retinitis, and vasculitis (exclude acute retinal necrosis)
  - Optic nerve hyperaemia or swelling (Figs. 14.1, 14.2, and 14.3)

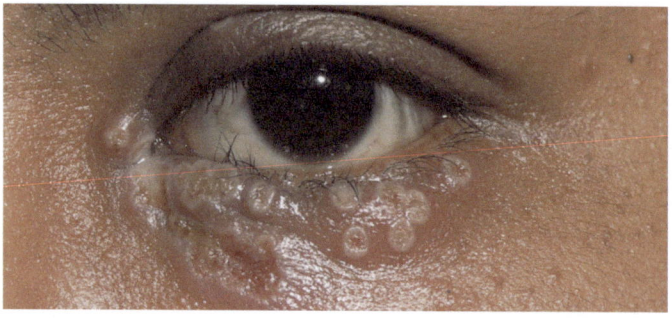

Fig. 14.1 Herpes zoster ophthalmicus (HZO). The photo depicts active vesicles on the lower lid margin of the left eye of this patient

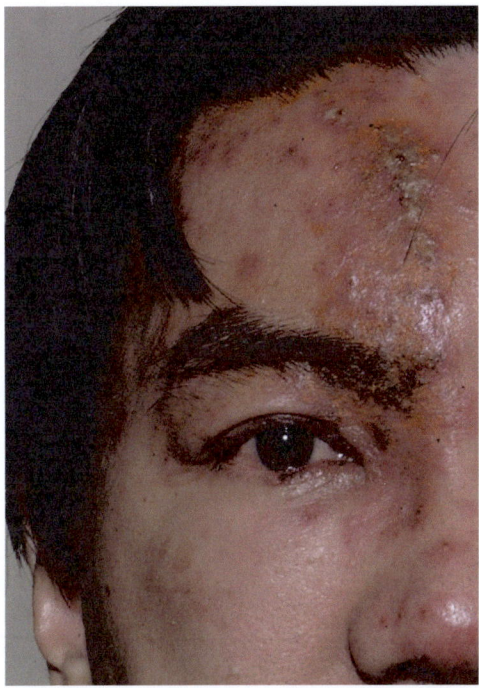

Fig. 14.2 This photo depicts a vesicular rash with crusting in the right V1 distribution including the tip of the nose (Hutchinson's sign) suggestive of right herpes zoster ophthalmicus (HZO)

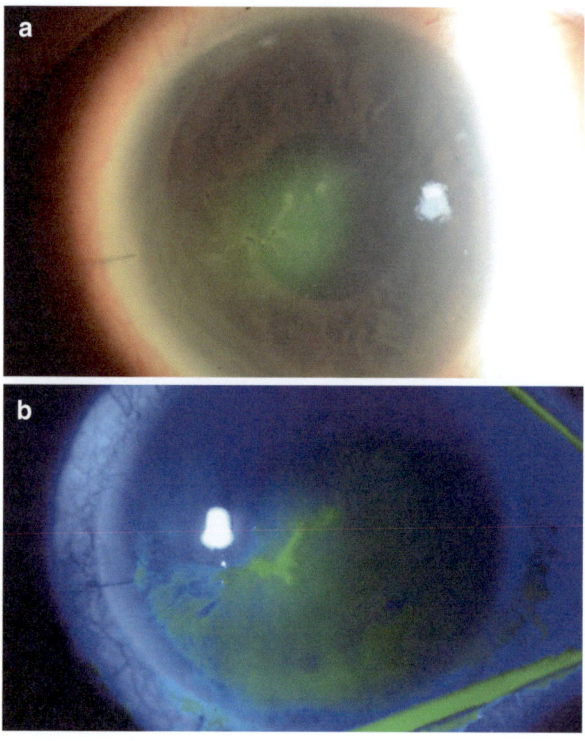

Fig. 14.3 (**a**, **b**) This patient underwent an endothelial keratoplasty with suture still in situ. There is an overlying central pseudo dendritic lesion with branching pattern with no terminal bulbs seen on fluorescein staining (normal beam on top, cobalt blue filter on bottom)

Investigations

- Consider HIV screen in young patients (<40 years old)

Treatment

- Oral acyclovir 800 mg 5×/day for 7–10 days (adjust in renal impairment)

- Topical acyclovir 5% ointment to facial vesicles
- Anterior uveitis or conjunctivitis present:
  - Topical acyclovir 3% ointment and steroids
- Corneal epithelial pseudodendrites present:
  - Topical acyclovir 3% ointment and antibiotics
  - Omit topical steroids
- Glaucoma drops if raised IOP
- Review patient after 1 week to watch for possible onset of uveitis
- Ask about and treat post-herpetic neuralgia
  - Analgesia: paracetamol, NSAIDs as first line
  - Consider gabapentin
- Referral to neurology and infectious disease in cases with cranial nerve palsies TRO intracranial spread and secondary complications, e.g. encephalitis
- Referral to infectious disease for HIV+ cases

GEH Perspectives
- *Be Aware of Eye Involvement*: Keep in mind that HZO can affect most structures of the eye. A thorough examination is essential to identify all possible complications.
- *Watch for Complications*: Cranial nerve palsies and elevated intraocular pressure (IOP) are common with HZO, so be vigilant for these signs. Early detection and management can prevent further complications.
- *Understand the Disease Progression*: In the first week of HZO, you'll typically see epithelial disease with pseudodendrites. By the second week, uveitis often develops. Monitoring these changes can help guide treatment.
- *Educate Patients on Post-Herpetic Neuralgia*: Inform patients that post-herpetic neuralgia can last for weeks or even months. Setting realistic expectations can help them cope better with this potential outcome.

Open Access This chapter is licensed under the terms of the Creative Commons Attribution-NonCommercial-NoDerivatives 4.0 International License (http://creativecommons.org/licenses/by-nc-nd/4.0/), which permits any non-commercial use, sharing, distribution and reproduction in any medium or format, as long as you give appropriate credit to the original author(s) and the source, provide a link to the Creative Commons license and indicate if you modified the licensed material. You do not have permission under this license to share adapted material derived from this chapter or parts of it.

The images or other third party material in this chapter are included in the chapter's Creative Commons license, unless indicated otherwise in a credit line to the material. If material is not included in the chapter's Creative Commons license and your intended use is not permitted by statutory regulation or exceeds the permitted use, you will need to obtain permission directly from the copyright holder.

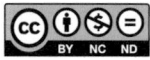

Chemical Injury

Nicole Sie, Marcus Ang, and Anshu Arundhati

Commence irrigation immediately!

History

- Type and amount of chemical—acid or alkali
- Time and mechanism of injury
- On-site eye irrigation
- Symptoms
  - Pain and photophobia
  - Redness
  - Tearing
  - Blurring of vision

Examination

- VA + RAPD + IOP
- Conjunctiva: Injection, chemists, extent of conjunctival staining (%), limbal staining, and ischaemia

---

N. Sie · A. Arundhati
Singapore National Eye Centre, Singapore Eye Research Institute, Singapore, Singapore

M. Ang (✉)
Department of Cornea and External Eye, Singapore National Eye Centre, Singapore Eye Research Institute, Singapore, Singapore
e-mail: marcus.Ang@Singhealth.com.sg

- Remove all retained particulate matter (evert eyelids and sweep fornices to remove trapped chemicals/debris)
- Epithelial defect—rule out infiltrates and assess with fluorescein, record size
- Extent of cornea oedema and loss of corneal clarity
- Anterior chamber activity
- Classify extent according to the Dua classification for prognostication (Figs. 15.1 and 15.2)

Dua classification for ocular surface burns				
Grade	Prognosis	Clinical findings (clock hours of limbal involvement)	Conjunctival involvement	Analogue scale
I	Very good	0	0%	0/0%
II	Good	<3	<30%	0.1–3/1%–29.9%
III	Good	3–6	30%–50%	3.1–6/31%–50%
IV	Good to guarded	6–9	50%–75%	6.1–9/51%–75%
V	Guarded to poor	9–12	75%–100%	9.1–11.9/75.1%–99.9%
VI	Very poor	Total limbus (12)	100%	0.12%

Credits: Dua HS, King AJ, Joseph A. A new classification of ocular surface burns. Br J Ophthalmol. 2001;85:1379–83

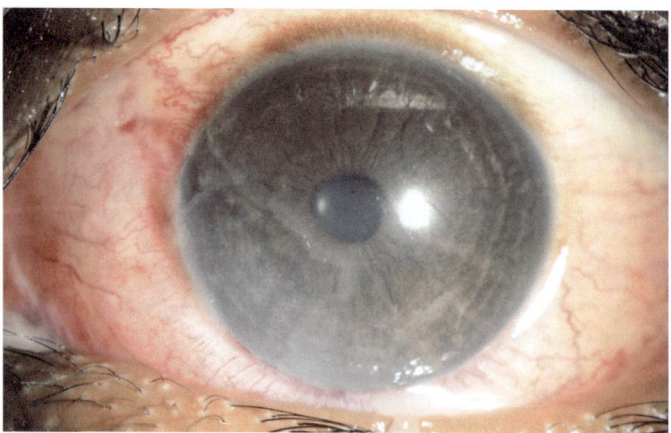

Fig. 15.1 This anterior segment photo depicts a patient who has sustained chemical injury. The conjunctiva is injected with limbal ischaemia nasally from 7 o'clock to 10 o'clock. There is a large epithelial defect nasally encroaching onto the visual axis

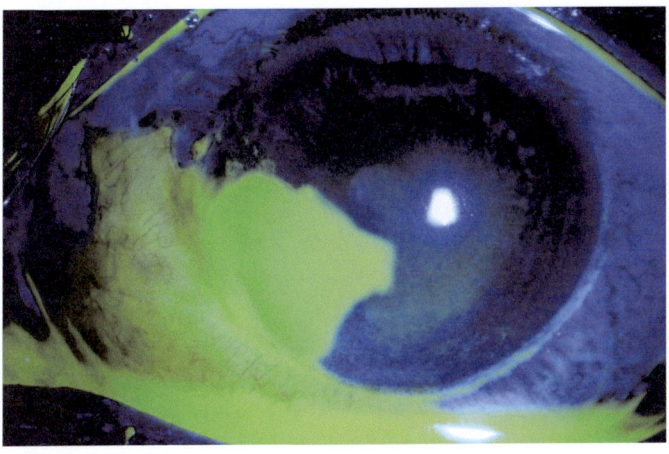

Fig. 15.2 This is the same eye as in Fig. 15.1, but with fluorescein staining showing the epithelial defect clearly, as well as conjunctival staining from 6 o'clock to 10 o'clock

Treatment

- Immediate management
  - Copious irrigation with saline or neutral solution for 30 min
  - Ensure fornix irrigation and remove particulate matter
  - Check pH after initial irrigation and continue irrigation until neutral (pH 7)
- Frequent preservative-free lubricants
- Topical antibiotics
- Topical preservative-free steroids
- ± Cycloplegic and analgesia
- ± Topical glaucoma medication for raised IOP
- ± Oral vitamin C 1000 mg and doxycycline
- Admission and daily review in severe cases

GEH Perspectives
- *Thoroughly Document Staining*: When assessing a chemical injury, be sure to document the extent of corneal and conjunctival staining carefully. Remember to check the fornices and evert the lids to get a comprehensive view of the injury's severity.
- *Look for Signs of Ischaemia*: Ischaemia might not be immediately obvious, so stay alert for subtle signs. Blanching of the vessels can be a helpful indicator of ischemia in the affected area, guiding your assessment and management decisions.

Open Access This chapter is licensed under the terms of the Creative Commons Attribution-NonCommercial-NoDerivatives 4.0 International License (http://creativecommons.org/licenses/by-nc-nd/4.0/), which permits any non-commercial use, sharing, distribution and reproduction in any medium or format, as long as you give appropriate credit to the original author(s) and the source, provide a link to the Creative Commons license and indicate if you modified the licensed material. You do not have permission under this license to share adapted material derived from this chapter or parts of it.

The images or other third party material in this chapter are included in the chapter's Creative Commons license, unless indicated otherwise in a credit line to the material. If material is not included in the chapter's Creative Commons license and your intended use is not permitted by statutory regulation or exceeds the permitted use, you will need to obtain permission directly from the copyright holder.

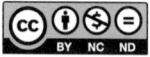

Bullous Keratopathy

Nicole Sie, Marcus Ang, and Anshu Arundhati

History

- Previous ocular lasers or surgeries and any complications
- Previous trauma, chemical injury
- Family history of corneal diseases
- Symptoms and duration
  - Classically patients may report blurring of vision—worse in morning

Examination

- VA, IOP
- RAPD (to prognosticate)
- Cornea:
  - Guttata, bullae, epithelial microcysts
  - Stain for epithelial defect
  - Descemet membrane folds/detachment

N. Sie · A. Arundhati
Singapore National Eye Centre, Singapore Eye Research Institute, Singapore, Singapore

M. Ang (✉)
Department of Cornea and External Eye, Singapore National Eye Centre, Singapore Eye Research Institute, Singapore, Singapore
e-mail: marcus.Ang@Singhealth.com.sg

- Scarring or neovascularisation
- Gonioscopy: retained lens material
- Previous posterior capsule rupture with vitreous endothelial touch
- Lens status: aphakia, pseudophakia, dense cataract, any subluxation/dislocation/secondary lens fixation
- Previous laser iridotomy, glaucoma filtration/tube surgery
- Signs of previous or active uveitis: anterior chamber inflammation, keratitis precipitates
- Dilated fundus examination: glaucoma, previous retinal detachment surgery, other retinal pathology (Figs. 16.1 and 16.2)

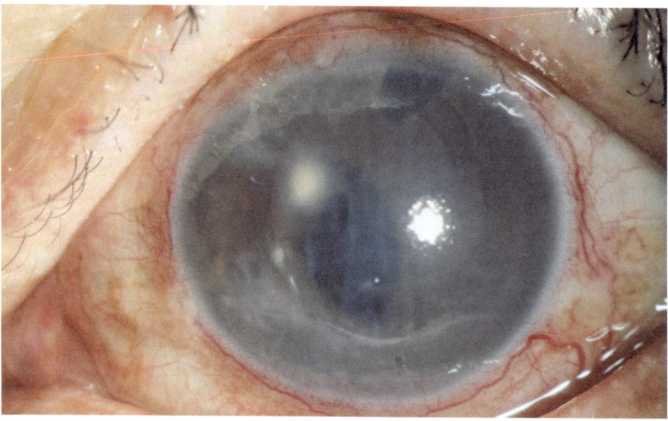

Fig. 16.1 This anterior segment photo shows a diffusely hazy cornea with Descemet's membrane folds with a corectopic pupil. There is also an anterior chamber IOL (ACIOL) with a patent superior peripheral iridectomy (PI)

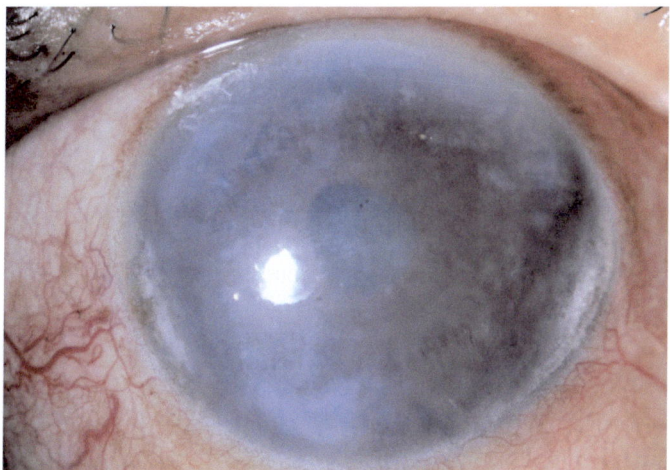

Fig. 16.2 This anterior segment photo shows a diffusely hazy cornea in a phakic patient

Investigations

- Cornea slit-lamp photographs
- Endothelial cell count
- Central corneal thickness
- Anterior segment OCT
- Corneal tomography
- B-scan U/S if no view of fundus

Treatment

- Management depends on visual potential, impact on vision and ADLs, and the presence of pain
- Treat underlying cause: repositioning or exchange of IOL if ACIOL/subluxated/dislocated, removal of retained lens fragment(s), treat active uveitis or elevated IOP

- Good visual potential
  - Conservative: lubricants, hypertonic saline, topical antibiotics for epithelial defect, treat overlying infection, consider bandage contact lens to prevent epithelial breakdown, control secondary inflammation
  - Surgical: endothelial keratoplasty
- Poor visual potential and no pain: conservative management as above
- Poor visual potential and pain: Gunderson flap

GEH Perspectives
Causes of bullous keratopathy

- Primary endothelial disease
  - Fuchs endothelial dystrophy
  - Iridocorneal endothelial syndrome
  - Anterior segment dysgenesis
- Secondary endothelial damage
  - Surgery (previous cataract surgery, aphakia, glaucoma surgery, laser peripheral iridotomy)
  - Trauma/chemical injury
  - Uveitis (long standing inflammation)/infection (Cytomegalovirus or herpes simplex virus) viral endotheliitis
  - Pressure (IOP high or low, uncontrolled glaucoma)

Open Access This chapter is licensed under the terms of the Creative Commons Attribution-NonCommercial-NoDerivatives 4.0 International License (http://creativecommons.org/licenses/by-nc-nd/4.0/), which permits any noncommercial use, sharing, distribution and reproduction in any medium or format, as long as you give appropriate credit to the original author(s) and the source, provide a link to the Creative Commons license and indicate if you modified the licensed material. You do not have permission under this license to share adapted material derived from this chapter or parts of it.

The images or other third party material in this chapter are included in the chapter's Creative Commons license, unless indicated otherwise in a credit line to the material. If material is not included in the chapter's Creative Commons license and your intended use is not permitted by statutory regulation or exceeds the permitted use, you will need to obtain permission directly from the copyright holder.

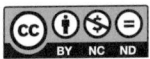

Corneal Graft Rejection

Nicole Sie and Marcus Ang

History

- Type of graft: full thickness or partial thickness
- Date of surgery
- Previous grafts and rejection episodes
- Previous viral infections
- Current medications and compliance (steroids, antibiotics, and glaucoma drops)
- Underlying primary pathology (e.g. Fuchs endothelial dystrophy)
- Ocular trauma
- Symptoms
  - Blurring of vision
  - Pain and photophobia
  - Redness
  - Tearing

N. Sie
Singapore National Eye Centre, Singapore Eye Research Institute, Singapore, Singapore

M. Ang (✉)
Department of Cornea and External Eye, Singapore National Eye Centre, Singapore Eye Research Institute, Singapore, Singapore
e-mail: marcus.Ang@Singhealth.com.sg

© The Authors(s) 2026
A. C S Tan et al. (eds.), *The Global Eye Health Handbook*,
https://doi.org/10.1007/978-981-96-8861-6_17

Examination

- VA and IOP
- Conjunctival injection
- Cornea
    - Subepithelial infiltrates (Krachmer spots)
    - Rejection line
    - Vascularization
    - Oedema
    - Sutures—loose/any infiltrate
    - Corneal endothelium—keratic precipitates (KP), Khodadoust line—rejection line
- AC flare and cells (Figs. 17.1 and 17.2)

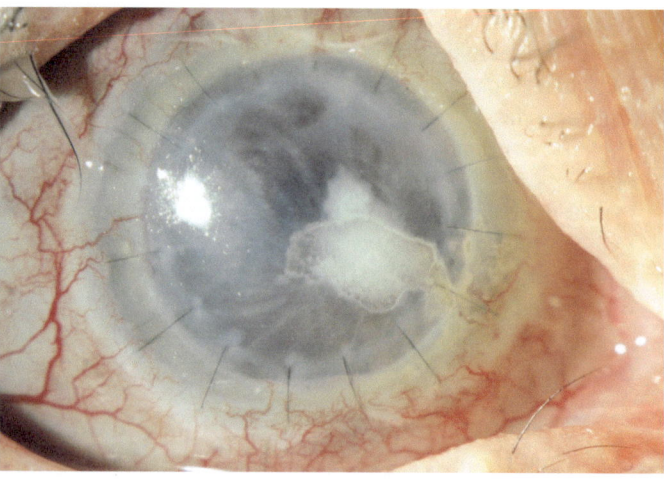

Fig. 17.1 This anterior segment photo illustrates a patient with a failed penetrating keratoplasty (PK). The sutures are intact, but the graft is diffusely hazy with a large central opacity with chronic secondary calcium deposition and deep corneal vascularisation

17 Corneal Graft Rejection

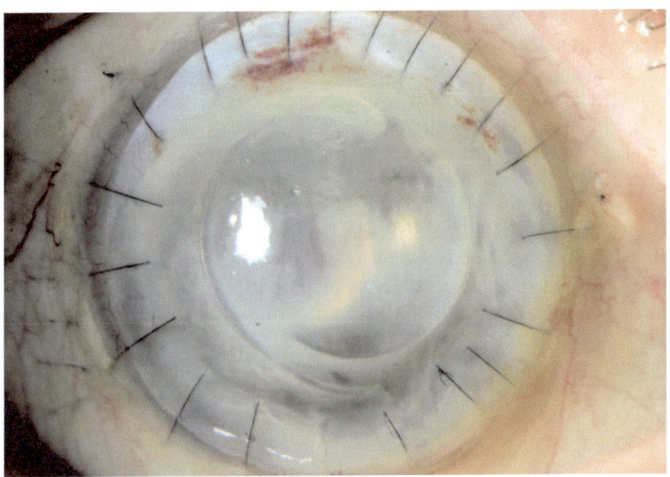

Fig. 17.2 Failed penetrating keratoplasty (PKP). This anterior segment photo shows an opacified graft with an anterior chamber intraocular lens

Treatment

- Inform primary corneal surgeon and corneal fellow
- Intensive topical steroids with antibiotic cover
- Review patient in a few hours/next day

> **GEH Perspectives**
> - Classic signs of rejection: Khodadoust line is only seen in penetrating keratoplasty.
> - Endothelial keratoplasty—signs are more subtle—with few KPs, localised oedema and minimal AC activity. Also consider cytomegalovirus (CMV) endotheliitis as a differential if stellate KPs, iris changes or not responding to treatment with topical steroids.
> - Anterior lamellar keratoplasty—only stromal and epithelial rejection occurs.
> - Check for compliance with medications.

Open Access This chapter is licensed under the terms of the Creative Commons Attribution-NonCommercial-NoDerivatives 4.0 International License (http://creativecommons.org/licenses/by-nc-nd/4.0/), which permits any noncommercial use, sharing, distribution and reproduction in any medium or format, as long as you give appropriate credit to the original author(s) and the source, provide a link to the Creative Commons license and indicate if you modified the licensed material. You do not have permission under this license to share adapted material derived from this chapter or parts of it.

The images or other third party material in this chapter are included in the chapter's Creative Commons license, unless indicated otherwise in a credit line to the material. If material is not included in the chapter's Creative Commons license and your intended use is not permitted by statutory regulation or exceeds the permitted use, you will need to obtain permission directly from the copyright holder.

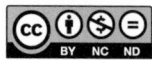

Infections: Blebitis

Claire Peterson, Zhu Li Yap, Sahil Thakur, and Rahat Husain

Introduction to Glaucoma

Glaucoma is a silent and chronic condition and is a major cause of irreversible blindness worldwide. Screening, treating, and long-term management of glaucoma can be challenging, especially in low-middle income countries.

Glaucoma Emergencies

The glaucoma emergencies detailed above are essential for any general ophthalmologist to know how to manage. However, in resource-limited settings or areas with restricted access to medications, laser equipment, or operating theatres, these tools may not always be readily available.

In the event of an emergency, it is important to administer prompt treatment. Patients can first be treated with maximum-

---

C. Peterson · Z. L. Yap (✉) · S. Thakur · R. Husain
Singapore National Eye Centre, Singapore Eye Research Institute, Singapore, Singapore
e-mail: yap.zhu.li@singhealth.com.sg

tolerated medical therapy until they are able to seek help at a larger eye centre.

- Acute high IOP
    - Suggested in the case of a painful red eye, mid-dilated pupil, hazy cornea
    - Eye will also feel hard on palpation through the eyelid, compared to the other eye
    - If IV medication is not available, first treat the patient with the maximum tolerable dose of oral acetazolamide (with oral potassium and bicarbonate replacement) along with anti-glaucoma eye drops before promptly referring them to an ophthalmic centre
- Infections
    - If suspected, swab (if possible), then treat patient with broad-spectrum topical antibiotics
    - Ensure the patient has no systemic infections—fever, chills, and rigours
    - Avoid starting steroids if the cause is unknown as steroids will exacerbate infections

Glaucoma Treatment

We often take a stepwise approach to treating glaucoma, with drops or lasers offered as first-line therapy before offering surgery. Additionally, patients with asymptomatic PACS also have the option of observation instead of LPI.

However, in areas with limited resources, this treatment paradigm may change due to challenges related to the affordability of eye drops and accessibility of care.

It may be more cost-effective to treat patients with a laser machine versus using long-term eye drops, as eye drops are expensive and may also have specific storage requirements. As found in the LiGHT trial, SLT is a safe treatment for OAG and OHT and provides better long-term disease control than initial eye drop therapy.

Screening

Screening programs are important as they can detect glaucoma before patients are symptomatic. This is important in glaucoma, where patients often already have significant irreversible vision loss by the time they are symptomatic.

Utilising technology to screen for glaucoma can be beneficial in regions with limited trained ophthalmic manpower. For example, a technician can be trained to capture fundus photos for screening, which can then be graded using artificial intelligence, allowing glaucoma suspects to be referred to the ophthalmic service for further evaluation.

Prompt Referral

Having safe and standardised referral pathways is crucial in managing glaucoma. In more resource-rich environments, we often rely on tests such as HVF testing and OCT measurements of the RNFL to screen and monitor for glaucomatous changes. However, these machines can be expensive and may not be readily accessible in many regions. Below is a suggested referral pathway adapted for the global eye health setting.

Patient Education

Last but not least, it is important to educate patients on the importance of eye screening, eye health, and common eye conditions. In our digital age, almost everyone has access or knows of someone with access to a smartphone. This allows us to easily distribute material digitally—through online flyers, videos, etc. Patient education initiatives should be supported by the local healthcare practitioners and in the patient's own native language or dialect.

History

- Date and indication for surgery
- Pain, redness, discharge
- Type of Glaucoma surgery, antimetabolite (MMC/5-FU) use

Examination

- VA and *RAPD*
- IOP
- Lid margin disease, e.g. blepharitis
- No more than trace anterior chamber (AC) cells and flare
- Absence of vitritis

Bleb Features

- Conjunctival injection with a white avascular bleb, giving a "white-on-red" appearance
- Infection risk: thin-walled, cystic, avascular
- Bleb content
- Location of bleb
- Seidel's test for bleb leak
- Loose sutures, presence of infiltrate

Investigations

- Ultrasound B-scan to exclude presence of vitritis
- Peri-bleb conjunctival swab
  - Gram stain
  - Culture plates: blood agar, chocolate agar, brain heart infusion broth
- Bleb photographs

Treatment

- Inform glaucoma fellow on-call and primary surgeon
- Cefazolin preservative free and gentamicin preservative free hourly until moxifloxacin is available
- Cycloplegics: atropine 1% three times a day
- Oral ciprofloxacin 500 mg twice a day
- Trace Gram stain and review 6 h later to assess pain, chemosis, AC activity, RAPD and VA
- If worse, repeat B scan, consider treatment for endophthalmitis
- If stable or better, review 24 h later, trace cultures (Figs. 18.1 and 18.2)

> **GEH Perspectives**
> - Blebitis typically presents with a white-on-red appearance

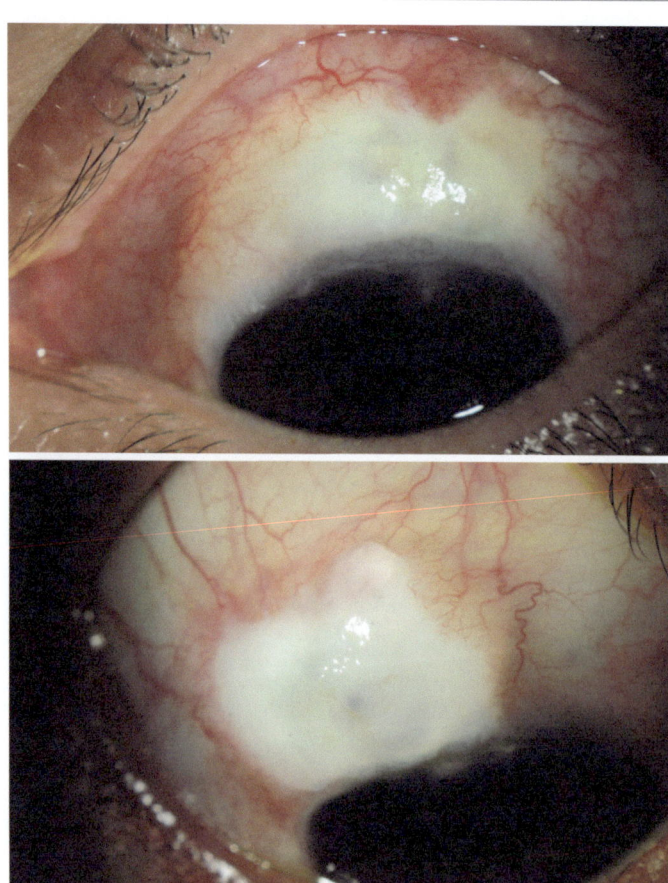

Figs. 18.1 and 18.2 The above anterior segment photos depict a superior cystic, thin-walled, avascular bleb with a "white-on-red" appearance, suggestive of blebitis

Open Access This chapter is licensed under the terms of the Creative Commons Attribution-NonCommercial-NoDerivatives 4.0 International License (http://creativecommons.org/licenses/by-nc-nd/4.0/), which permits any noncommercial use, sharing, distribution and reproduction in any medium or format, as long as you give appropriate credit to the original author(s) and the source, provide a link to the Creative Commons license and indicate if you modified the licensed material. You do not have permission under this license to share adapted material derived from this chapter or parts of it.

The images or other third party material in this chapter are included in the chapter's Creative Commons license, unless indicated otherwise in a credit line to the material. If material is not included in the chapter's Creative Commons license and your intended use is not permitted by statutory regulation or exceeds the permitted use, you will need to obtain permission directly from the copyright holder.

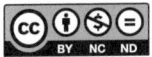

Infections: Bleb-Related Endophthalmitis

Claire Peterson, Zhu Li Yap, Sahil Thakur, and Rahat Husain

History

- Date and indication for surgery
- Pain, redness, and discharge
- BOV

Examination

- VA and *RAPD*
- IOP
- Intense AC inflammation and/or hypopyon, and/or vitritis
- Lid margin disease, e.g. MGD (*risk factor*)

Bleb Features

- Conjunctival injection with "white-on-red" bleb appearance
- Thin-walled cystic avascular bleb
- Location of bleb
- Seidel test
- Loose sutures, infiltrates

C. Peterson · Z. L. Yap (✉) · S. Thakur · R. Husain
Singapore National Eye Centre, Singapore Eye Research Institute, Singapore, Singapore
e-mail: yap.zhu.li@singhealth.com.sg

Investigations

- B-scan if no view of posterior segment
- Peri-bleb conjunctival swab for Gram stain, blood agar, chocolate agar, and BHIB
- Vitreous tap (as above)

Treatment

- Inform primary surgeon and refer to glaucoma and vitreo-retina service
- Admit
- Intravitreal vancomycin and ceftazidime (as for post-operative endophthalmitis)
- Topical antibiotics (as for blebitis)
- Atropine 1% three times a day
- Oral ciprofloxacin 500 mg twice a day
- Keep in view vitrectomy for diagnostic/therapeutic reasons
- Trace Gram stain urgently and assess clinical progress
- ± Refer Infectious Disease Team

> **GEH Perspectives**
> - *Keep Bleb-Related Endophthalmitis (BRE) in Mind*: Always consider bleb-related endophthalmitis in any case of blebitis with more than trace anterior chamber cells. Early suspicion can make a big difference in outcomes.
> - *Act Quickly*: Bleb-related infections tend to progress faster than post-cataract surgery endophthalmitis. It is important to have a low threshold for performing a vitrectomy when managing suspected bleb-related endophthalmitis (BRE) to prevent rapid deterioration.

Open Access This chapter is licensed under the terms of the Creative Commons Attribution-NonCommercial-NoDerivatives 4.0 International License (http://creativecommons.org/licenses/by-nc-nd/4.0/), which permits any noncommercial use, sharing, distribution and reproduction in any medium or format, as long as you give appropriate credit to the original author(s) and the source, provide a link to the Creative Commons license and indicate if you modified the licensed material. You do not have permission under this license to share adapted material derived from this chapter or parts of it.

The images or other third party material in this chapter are included in the chapter's Creative Commons license, unless indicated otherwise in a credit line to the material. If material is not included in the chapter's Creative Commons license and your intended use is not permitted by statutory regulation or exceeds the permitted use, you will need to obtain permission directly from the copyright holder.

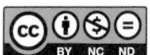

Acute Angle Closure

20

Claire Peterson, Zhu Li Yap, Sahil Thakur, and Rahat Husain

History

- Duration of symptoms
- Ocular trauma
- Previous episodes with similar symptoms
- Symptoms
- Pain, redness, and tearing
- Nausea, vomiting and headache
- Blurring of vision
- Lens-induced glaucoma may have a history of progressive blurring of vision

Examination

- Conjunctival injection
- Corneal oedema
- AC shallowing with cells and flare
- Cataract (may be white, intumescent, hypermature, or subluxated)

C. Peterson · Z. L. Yap (✉) · S. Thakur · R. Husain
Singapore National Eye Centre, Singapore Eye Research Institute, Singapore, Singapore
e-mail: yap.zhu.li@singhealth.com.sg

- Raised IOP
- Fixed and mid-dilated (check RAPD by reverse method)
- Attempt gonioscopy—ideally 4-mirror Sussman dynamic gonioscopy

Investigations

- Renal panel
- ECG and chest X-ray
- Weight (if mannitol required)
- U/S B-scan if no view of posterior segment
- Ultrasound biomicroscopy and preoperative workup for lens-induced glaucoma

Treatment (APAC)

- Intravenous Acetazolamide 500 mg
- Topical Alphagan, Timolol, Latanoprost, Pred Forte (5 min between drops)
- Recheck IOP 90 min after intravenous acetazolamide
- IOP still high → second dose acetazolamide 500 mg

When IOP is better, with clear cornea:

- Pilocarpine 2% to attack eye (to be used when IOP <30) and 2% to fellow eye (Pilo 4% not currently available)
- Laser peripheral iridotomy (LPI) to attack eye and fellow eye (can wait until next day if IOP is <30 mmHg)
- Discharge with Pred Forte three hourly, glaucoma drops
- Follow-up at glaucoma clinic in 1–3 days to check IOP and LPI patency
- Keep on oral acetazolamide a few days post-laser
- IOP better but still with significant corneal oedema → contact glaucoma fellow to arrange next-day follow-up
- Consider phacoemulsification within 1 week of acute attack instead of performing an LPI if experienced cataract surgeon is present

GEH Perspectives
- *Always examine the fellow eye as it should also be shallow with narrow angles in APAC; if not, consider other diagnoses of secondary angle closure.*
  - In the setting of APAC, patients should be given miotics after reduction of IOP to prepare them for a LPI (definitive treatment of pupil block).
  - Secondary angle closure (e.g. lens-induced) will benefit from Atropine instead of Pilocarpine.

Do not "pulse" anti-glaucoma medications, just administer a stat dose and as prescribed.

Open Access This chapter is licensed under the terms of the Creative Commons Attribution-NonCommercial-NoDerivatives 4.0 International License (http://creativecommons.org/licenses/by-nc-nd/4.0/), which permits any noncommercial use, sharing, distribution and reproduction in any medium or format, as long as you give appropriate credit to the original author(s) and the source, provide a link to the Creative Commons license and indicate if you modified the licensed material. You do not have permission under this license to share adapted material derived from this chapter or parts of it.

The images or other third party material in this chapter are included in the chapter's Creative Commons license, unless indicated otherwise in a credit line to the material. If material is not included in the chapter's Creative Commons license and your intended use is not permitted by statutory regulation or exceeds the permitted use, you will need to obtain permission directly from the copyright holder.

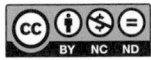

Neovascular Glaucoma

Claire Peterson, Zhu Li Yap, Sahil Thakur, and Rahat Husain

History

- Duration of symptoms
- History of ischemic retinal disease (central retinal vein occlusion, proliferative diabetic retinopathy, and ocular ischemic syndrome [OIS])
- Vascular risk factors (diabetes, hypertension, and ischemic heart disease)
- Eye pain, redness, and tearing
- Nausea, vomiting, and headache
- Blurring of vision

Examination

- Conjunctival injection
- Corneal oedema
- AC cells, flare, and neovascularization of iris (NVI)
- Gonioscopy showing neovascularisation of angle and peripheral anterior synechiae

---

C. Peterson · Z. L. Yap (✉) · S. Thakur · R. Husain
Singapore National Eye Centre, Singapore Eye Research Institute, Singapore, Singapore
e-mail: yap.zhu.li@singhealth.com.sg

- High IOP
- Dilated fundoscopy to determine cause
- Auscultation for carotid bruit

Investigations

- Ultrasound B-scan if retina not visible
- Capillary glucose and BP
- Renal panel, CXR, ECG, and weight (if mannitol required)
- Carotid ultrasound and cardiac echocardiogram for OIS

Treatment

- Intravenous acetazolamide 500 mg—confirm no renal dysfunction (more common in NVG patients)
- Topical Timolol and Alphagan (second line: latanoprost, intravenous mannitol)
- Atropine 1% three times a day
- Topical steroids
- Refer to retina service for management of underlying cause (e.g. panretinal photocoagulation, anti-vascular endothelial growth factor)
- Refer to glaucoma service for follow-up
- Co-manage underlying medical conditions with a physician (Fig. 21.1)

21 Neovascular Glaucoma

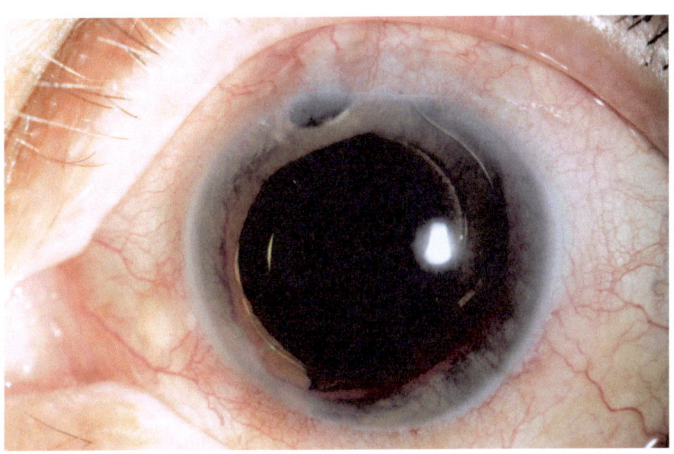

Fig. 21.1 This anterior segment photo shows an anterior chamber supported intraocular lens with frank new vessels at the iris, with a hyphaema

> **GEH Perspectives**
> - *Dual Approach to Treatment*: Managing NVG involves addressing both the elevated intraocular pressure (glaucoma) and the underlying cause—usually retinal ischemia. Treating both is key to better outcomes.
> - *Assess the Bigger Picture*: When planning treatment, consider the patient's visual prognosis, any pain they may be experiencing, and the condition of the fellow eye. This helps guide whether aggressive treatment or more conservative care is the best approach.
> - *Focus on Quality of Life*: In cases with poor visual prognosis or significant pain, prioritize treatments that maintain comfort and preserve the patient's quality of life.

Open Access This chapter is licensed under the terms of the Creative Commons Attribution-NonCommercial-NoDerivatives 4.0 International License (http://creativecommons.org/licenses/by-nc-nd/4.0/), which permits any non-commercial use, sharing, distribution and reproduction in any medium or format, as long as you give appropriate credit to the original author(s) and the source, provide a link to the Creative Commons license and indicate if you modified the licensed material. You do not have permission under this license to share adapted material derived from this chapter or parts of it.

The images or other third party material in this chapter are included in the chapter's Creative Commons license, unless indicated otherwise in a credit line to the material. If material is not included in the chapter's Creative Commons license and your intended use is not permitted by statutory regulation or exceeds the permitted use, you will need to obtain permission directly from the copyright holder.

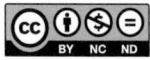

Lens-Induced Glaucoma

22

Claire Peterson, Zhu Li Yap, Sahil Thakur, and Shamira Perera

History

- Trauma
- Family history of glaucoma
- Previous surgeries
- Symptoms and duration
- Pain
- Blurring of vision—changes with position
- Redness

Examination

- VA, IOP, RAPD (by reverse method if fixed and dilated)
- Fellow eye (asymmetry of AC depth)
- Slit lamp examination: corneal clarity, phacodonesis, subluxation or dislocation, any vitreous in AC (± iris/cornea touch)
- Gonioscopy

C. Peterson · Z. L. Yap (✉) · S. Thakur · S. Perera
Singapore National Eye Centre, Singapore Eye Research Institute, Singapore, Singapore
e-mail: yap.zhu.li@singhealth.com.sg

Investigations

- B-scan to assess retinal status if poor view
- Ultrasound biomicroscopy, if available
- Place patient in supine position and assess if lens falls back

Treatment

- Ocular emergency requiring urgent reduction of IOP to clear cornea for subsequent definitive cataract surgery
- Acute medical management of IOP: Intravenous acetazolamide 500 mg, failing which intravenous mannitol 20% 0.5–2 g/kg in absence of contraindications, topical glaucoma medications
- Topical steroids
- Atropine
- Lay patient supine
- Once cornea is clear and IOP is controlled, arrange for early cataract surgery
  - If lens is dislocated: management depends on location, patient, and ocular factors
    - Anterior dislocation into AC: ocular emergency, requires immediate surgical removal (lens explanation)
    - Posterior dislocation into vitreous
      (a) Lens capsule intact with no inflammation: consider leaving in situ
      (b) Lens capsule breached with inflammation: trans pars plana vitrectomy (TPPV)/lensectomy

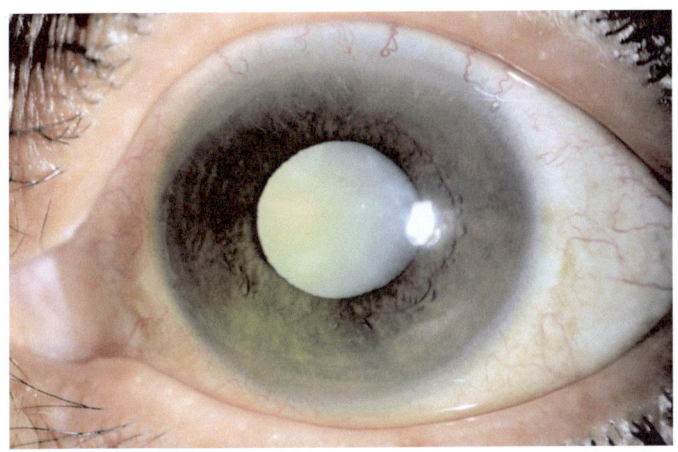

This anterior segment photo shows an intumescent white cataract

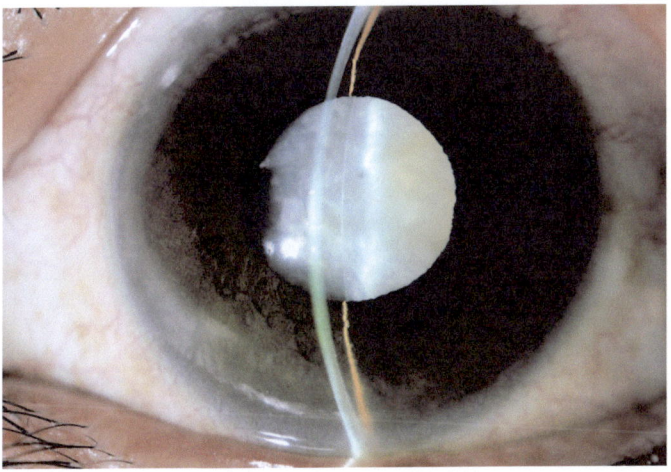

This anterior segment photo shows the slit beam demonstrating a shallow anterior chamber with an intumescent white cataract

> **GEH Perspectives**
> Closed angle
>
> - Phacomorphic: Intumescent lens causing pupil block
> - Subluxed lens: Anterior lens displacement causing pupil block
>
> Open angle
>
> - Phacolytic: Hyper mature cataract causing leakage of lens proteins through intact capsule
> - Phacoantigenic: Autoimmune granulomatous reaction to exposed lens proteins from *ruptured* capsule
> - Lens particle glaucoma: Retained lens fragments obstruct trabecular meshwork

Open Access This chapter is licensed under the terms of the Creative Commons Attribution-NonCommercial-NoDerivatives 4.0 International License (http://creativecommons.org/licenses/by-nc-nd/4.0/), which permits any non-commercial use, sharing, distribution and reproduction in any medium or format, as long as you give appropriate credit to the original author(s) and the source, provide a link to the Creative Commons license and indicate if you modified the licensed material. You do not have permission under this license to share adapted material derived from this chapter or parts of it.

The images or other third party material in this chapter are included in the chapter's Creative Commons license, unless indicated otherwise in a credit line to the material. If material is not included in the chapter's Creative Commons license and your intended use is not permitted by statutory regulation or exceeds the permitted use, you will need to obtain permission directly from the copyright holder.

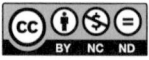

Acute Anterior Uveitis

23

Joshua Lim and Andrew Tsai

Introduction to Uveitis

1. Accurate Diagnosis
    It might be helpful to consider a few key points when managing ocular inflammation.
    (a) Establishing the type and location of inflammation through thorough history taking and clinical examination can guide an accurate diagnosis.
    (b) Understanding the general approach to differential diagnosis—starting with ruling out treatable infective causes, then inflammatory, and finally considering masquerade conditions—could also be useful.
    (c) Being aware of common infective and inflammatory causes in your geographic location might help in prioritising certain diagnoses over others.
2. Prompt and Effective Treatment
    (a) In terms of treatment, timely intervention is essential for uveitis patients to prevent complications like cataract formation, posterior synechiae, or intraocular pressure spikes.

J. Lim · A. Tsai (✉)
Singapore National Eye Centre, Singapore Eye Research Institute, Singapore, Singapore
e-mail: andrew.tsai.s.h@singhealth.com.sg

(b) It is important to remember that steroids, while useful, may not always be the right choice—especially when viral causes are involved—so careful use is advised.
(c) Having a reliable supply of essentials like topical corticosteroids, cycloplegics, and IOP-lowering agents, especially in smaller or remote locations, could make a big difference in patient care.
3. Referral and Specialist Care
   (a) Identifying complicated cases early and referring patients with severe, recurrent, or atypical uveitis to tertiary centres could be a helpful strategy.
   (b) Establishing strong referral pathways and networks with these centres can provide valuable support in managing challenging cases.
   (c) Tools like telemedicine or remote review of slit lamp photos and test results might also help reduce delays in treatment.
4. Reliable Documentation and Reporting
   (a) Keeping detailed records of patient notes and test results for ongoing monitoring.
   (b) Additionally, engaging in local research or collaborating with larger centres could offer valuable insights into the epidemiology of uveitis in your community and help refine treatment protocols over time.

History

Ocular Symptoms:

- Redness, pain, and photophobia
- Blurring of vision
- Floaters

Systemic Symptoms:

- Rashes
- Gastrointestinal symptoms with loss of appetite and weight
- Ulcers

- Medical history
- Immune status
- Underlying infections (e.g. tuberculosis (TB), syphilis)
- Connective tissue disease (e.g. ankylosing spondylitis, rheumatoid arthritis)

Examination

- Circumciliary injection
- Corneal oedema, infiltrates, reduced sensation
- AC activity (cells, flare, hypopyon, fibrin) and KPs
- Posterior synechiae
- Iris nodules (Busacca, Koeppe) and iris atrophy
- Raised IOP
- Vitritis, macular oedema, retinitis, vasculitis, or choroiditis
- Disc oedema or hyperaemia

Investigations (If Available)

- FBC, ESR, CRP
- Renal panel, liver panel, urine microscopy
- Chest X-ray
- Specific investigations
- Sacroiliac joint X-ray
- Mantoux test, T-spot TB, venereal disease research laboratory (VDRL), and syphilis line immunoassay (LIA)
- HLA-B27 genotyping
- AC paracentesis for tetraplex PCR in cases of Posner-Schlossmann syndrome and Fuchs Heterochromic Iridocyclitis (FHI)

Treatment

- Topical medications
- Steroids
- Cycloplegia (e.g. homatropine three times a day)

- NSAIDs and glaucoma medications for hypertensive uveitis
- Systemic medications
- Ibuprofen for episcleritis and scleritis
- Early review and referral to uveitis service for complex cases (Figs. 23.1 and 23.2)

> **GEH Perspectives**
> - Granulomatous KPs are often a harbinger of serious systemic illness and warrant prompt referral to a Uveitis service
> - Obtaining a comprehensive medical history is mandatory in all cases of new-onset anterior uveitis

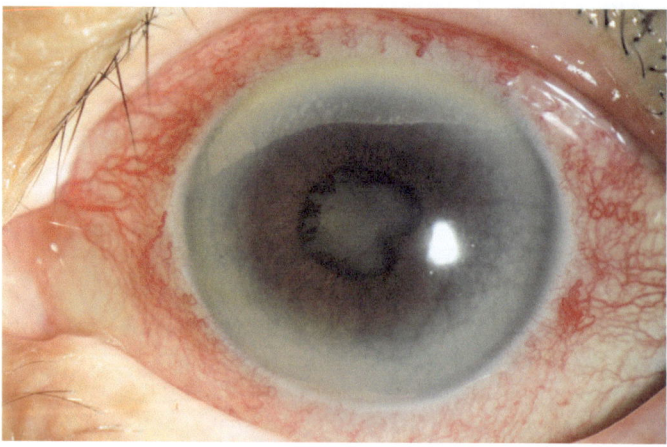

Fig. 23.1 This anterior segment photo shows circumciliary injection with an irregular pupil due to posterior synechiae (PS). There are some fresh non-pigmented keratic precipitates (KP) inferiorly. This patient has acute anterior uveitis (AAU)

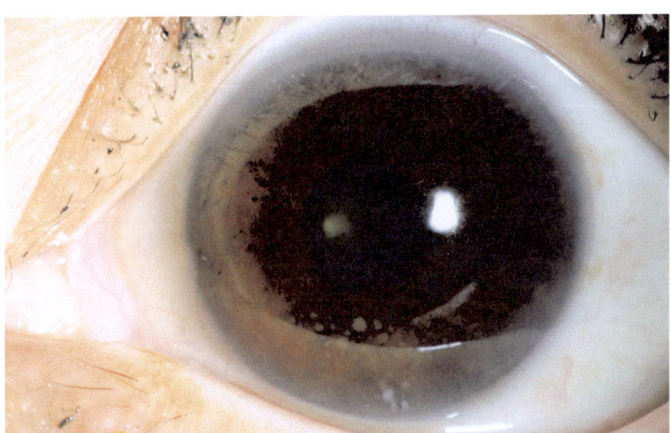

Fig. 23.2 This anterior segment photo shows granulomatous mutton-fat keratic precipitates on the cornea endothelium. The pupil is irregular with posterior synechiae (PS) at 3 o'clock and ectropion uveae

Open Access This chapter is licensed under the terms of the Creative Commons Attribution-NonCommercial-NoDerivatives 4.0 International License (http://creativecommons.org/licenses/by-nc-nd/4.0/), which permits any non-commercial use, sharing, distribution and reproduction in any medium or format, as long as you give appropriate credit to the original author(s) and the source, provide a link to the Creative Commons license and indicate if you modified the licensed material. You do not have permission under this license to share adapted material derived from this chapter or parts of it.

The images or other third party material in this chapter are included in the chapter's Creative Commons license, unless indicated otherwise in a credit line to the material. If material is not included in the chapter's Creative Commons license and your intended use is not permitted by statutory regulation or exceeds the permitted use, you will need to obtain permission directly from the copyright holder.

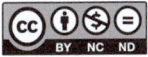

Infections: Orbital Cellulitis

24

Lim Xian Hui and Yvonne Chung

Introduction to Oculoplastics

- *Look at the patient and not just the eye*: As oculoplastic surgery conditions often involve areas around the eye, e.g. orbit, lacrimal gland, lacrimal drainage system, and eyelids, it is crucial that one takes a step back to look at the patient's face with a keen eye for detail, as signs of pathology can easily be missed if one were to focus only on performing an ocular examination.
- *Be thorough and meticulous*: Signs of pathology can be subtle, and abnormalities may sometimes be disguised by asymmetry with the fellow eye, e.g. appearance of ptosis in the normal eye due to lid retraction in the fellow eye. Furthermore, being a surgical subspecialty, good preoperative measurements and documentation (such as with photos) are required, as they can be used to plan surgical techniques and are necessary bulwarks in medicolegal cases.
- *Imaging, imaging, imaging*: Consider whether radiological scans are required, what question one is trying to answer with the scan, and which modality of imaging would yield the most helpful result. Computed Tomography (CT) scans are usually

L. X. Hui · Y. Chung (✉)
Singapore National Eye Centre, Singapore Eye Research Institute,
Singapore, Singapore
e-mail: chung.hsi.wei@singhealth.com.sg

faster and more affordable to obtain than Magnetic Resonance Imaging (MRI) scans. They are good for screening purposes or helping with assessing fractures and/or surgical planning due to its bone window. However, they entail exposure to radiation and cannot visualise soft tissue structures as well as MRI scans.
- *Is a tissue sample necessary?* Biopsies of suspicious lesions can help clinch a diagnosis quickly in many cases. Consider the type of biopsy that is required (e.g. shave vs. wedge resection, incisional vs. excisional), the approach that might be required to access the lesion (e.g. intra-orbital lesions) and how to close the wound nicely thereafter (e.g. skin tension lines). A close working relationship with the pathology colleagues reading the tissue sample slides can help one clarify possible diagnoses and inform of the need for closer monitoring in complicated or equivocal cases.

History

- Acute or subacute onset
- Periorbital pain, redness, swelling
- Diplopia or blurring of vision
- Fever, chills, and rigour (patient may appear toxic)
- History of sinusitis, dacryocystitis, periorbital skin trauma, insect bites, recent aesthetic procedure, chalazion, or dental infection (younger patients), headache
- Poorly controlled diabetes or immunocompromised (older patients)
- Previous eyelid/orbital surgery

Examination

- Vital signs (febrile, toxic)
- Reduced VA and colour vision, RAPD, visual fields
- Periorbital swelling, erythema, warmth +/− tenderness
- Raised IOP

24 Infections: Orbital Cellulitis

- Limited EOMs
- Pain on eye movements
- Proptosis (document with exophthalmometer if available), globe displacement
- Lagophthalmos and corneal staining
- Conjunctival injection and chemosis
- Disc swelling, retina vascular occlusion

Investigations

- Emergent CT orbit and paranasal sinus
- Look for possible cause of orbital cellulitis, exclude orbital/subperiosteal abscesses that require urgent drainage
- Full blood count and C-reactive protein
- Blood cultures
- Swab of conjunctival/wound discharge for aerobic culture, if present
- Preoperative workup if abscess is present and planned for urgent surgical drainage (CXR, ECG, PT/aPTT, renal panel)

Treatment

- Keep patient fasted
- Admit patient, inform consultant in charge/on call, refer to oculoplastic team
- Intravenous antibiotics (co-amoxiclav, cloxacillin +/− metronidazole)
- Topical antibiotics (levofloxacin eye drops)
- Analgesia
- Lubricants for corneal exposure/chemosis
- IOP-lowering eye drops, if necessary
- Close monitoring of optic nerve function initially
- ± Referral to otolaryngology, dentistry, or infectious disease team

Clinical Pearls

- Examine both eyes carefully and consider differential diagnosis of cavernous sinus thrombosis if infection is very severe and the patient appears to be very unwell and exhibits altered mental status and/or complex ophthalmoplegia.
- Be mindful of penicillin allergy—empiric antibiotics may need alteration.

GEH Perspectives
- *History and Exam Are Key*: Taking a careful history and performing a thorough clinical exam are essential in distinguishing preseptal cellulitis from orbital cellulitis. This distinction helps identify which patients might need further imaging, especially to look for abscesses that may need drainage, while also making sure resources are used wisely.
- *Imaging May Be a Challenge*: In some settings, access to radiological imaging might be limited. In these cases, your history and clinical examination might be the only way to decide whether the patient needs admission for intravenous antibiotics or if they can be treated as an outpatient with oral antibiotics.
- *Monitor Closely*: Orbital cellulitis can progress rapidly, so close monitoring of patients is essential. Pay special attention to vital signs and optic nerve function to assess their response to treatment, especially during the initial admission phase.
- *Avoid Overlooking Complications*: Secondary issues like corneal ulcers from exposure keratopathy, glaucoma from raised intraocular pressure, or compressive optic neuropathy can occur with orbital cellulitis and lead to long-term vision problems if not managed properly.
- *Know Your Pathogens*: Being aware of the common pathogens causing periorbital infections in your region can help guide effective antibiotic treatment, which is especially important in areas with endemic diseases.

- *Work as a Team*: Multidisciplinary care is often needed for these patients. For example, co-managing with an ENT team to drain sinus infections can be crucial in treating the underlying cause of the orbital cellulitis efficiently.

Open Access This chapter is licensed under the terms of the Creative Commons Attribution-NonCommercial-NoDerivatives 4.0 International License (http://creativecommons.org/licenses/by-nc-nd/4.0/), which permits any noncommercial use, sharing, distribution and reproduction in any medium or format, as long as you give appropriate credit to the original author(s) and the source, provide a link to the Creative Commons license and indicate if you modified the licensed material. You do not have permission under this license to share adapted material derived from this chapter or parts of it.

The images or other third party material in this chapter are included in the chapter's Creative Commons license, unless indicated otherwise in a credit line to the material. If material is not included in the chapter's Creative Commons license and your intended use is not permitted by statutory regulation or exceeds the permitted use, you will need to obtain permission directly from the copyright holder.

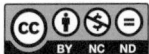

Infections: Dacryocystitis

Lim Xian Hui and Yvonne Chung

History

- Pain, redness, and swelling medial to eye and inferior to medial canthal tendon
- Purulent discharge from eye and/or skin fistula over localised swelling
- Previous similar episodes
- Fever, diplopia, blurring of vision
- Pre-existing tearing +/− discharge in eye, history of previous periorbital trauma/fractures/surgery
- Previous episodes of similar symptoms

Examination

- Vital signs especially temperature (suspect orbital cellulitis if febrile)
- Localised swelling and erythema with exquisite tenderness on palpation medial to eye and inferior to medial canthal tendon (lacrimal sac)

- Reflux of purulent discharge into eye on gentle pressure over inflamed lacrimal sac
- +/− associated cellulitis of surrounding periorbital skin
- +/− spontaneous discharging skin fistula from area of localised swelling
- Remove inflamed puncta
- Rule out complications such as orbital cellulitis (refer to previous chapter)

Investigations

- Conjunctival +/− skin swab of discharge for aerobic culture
- +/− CT orbits with contrast if unusual demographic or suspicion of complications (e.g. young patient, orbital cellulitis)

Treatment

- Refer to the oculoplastics team
- If orbital cellulitis or severe infection is refractory to previous oral antibiotic treatment, admit patient and follow pathway for orbital cellulitis
- Start systemic antibiotics—Oral co-amoxiclav +/− Cloxacillin
- Start topical antibiotics—Levofloxacin eye drops
- +/− PO Ibuprofen
- Analgesia
- +/− incision and drainage or aspiration of lacrimal sac abscess
- Syringing and dacryocystorhinostomy after acute infection have resolved

Clinical Pearls

- If there is a history of blood-stained tears—consider possibility of malignancy causing nasolacrimal duct obstruction

25 Infections: Dacryocystitis

GEH Perspectives
- *Confirm the Diagnosis*: In dacryocystitis, the swelling is usually located below the medial canthal tendon. If you notice swelling above this point, consider other possible diagnoses. Examining the puncti and canaliculi under the slit lamp is also key, as canaliculitis can present similarly but doesn't require a dacryocystorhinostomy (DCR) down the line.
- *Localize the Infection*: Gently pressing over the lacrimal drainage system while watching for purulent discharge from the puncti can help pinpoint the source of infection. This can be helpful in guiding treatment.
- *Rule Out Serious Causes*: Always keep malignancy in mind as a potential cause of nasolacrimal duct obstruction. Careful questioning and examination can help rule this out. If the patient is young or has a history that suggests secondary acquired nasolacrimal duct obstruction (e.g. facial trauma or malignancy), consider radiological imaging to confirm.
- *Consider Surgical Options*: Before deciding on surgery, think about the patient's overall condition, such as whether they are phakic or pseudophakic, their fitness for surgery and anaesthesia, and their personal preferences. For elderly patients, especially those who've had cataract surgery or those hesitant about surgery, prophylactic topical antibiotics might be a good alternative to improve quality of life without surgery.

Open Access This chapter is licensed under the terms of the Creative Commons Attribution-NonCommercial-NoDerivatives 4.0 International License (http://creativecommons.org/licenses/by-nc-nd/4.0/), which permits any noncommercial use, sharing, distribution and reproduction in any medium or format, as long as you give appropriate credit to the original author(s) and the source, provide a link to the Creative Commons license and indicate if you modified the licensed material. You do not have permission under this license to share adapted material derived from this chapter or parts of it.

The images or other third party material in this chapter are included in the chapter's Creative Commons license, unless indicated otherwise in a credit line to the material. If material is not included in the chapter's Creative Commons license and your intended use is not permitted by statutory regulation or exceeds the permitted use, you will need to obtain permission directly from the copyright holder.

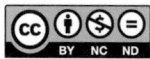

Carotid Cavernous Fistula (CCF)

Reuben Foo, Shweta Singhal, and Umapathi Thirugnanam

History

- Any significant head trauma/preceding intracranial or sinus surgery preceding onset of eye symptoms
- History of vascular risk factors especially hypertension
- Proptosis, chemosis, red eye—time of onset, acute vs. chronic
- Blurring of vision, diplopia, ptosis
- Pulsatile tinnitus, headache

Examination

- **Key clinical signs:**
- Conjunctival injection/corkscrew vessels/chemosis
- In early cases to distinguish from conjunctivitis look for the following red flags:
  - Raised intraocular pressure (+/− pulsatile mires in applanation tonometry)
  - Signs of optic neuropathy (reduced VA with RAPD and reduced colour vision)

R. Foo · S. Singhal (✉) · U. Thirugnanam
Singapore National Eye Centre, Singapore Eye Research Institute, Singapore, Singapore
e-mail: shweta.singhal@singhealth.com.sg

- Limited ocular motility, cranial nerve III, IV, V1/V2, VI palsies +/− Horner's syndrome
- Proptosis
• In advanced cases the following may also be present:
  - Ocular bruit
  - Exposure keratopathy
  - Anterior segment ischaemia (if chronic)
  - Disc swelling, ischaemic optic neuropathy
  - Dilated retinal veins, central retinal vein occlusion, choroidal detachment

Direct CCF clinical manifestations are usually severe. Indirect CCFs can be mild or asymptomatic.

Investigations

- Ideally MRI brain and orbits with contrast and MR Angiography
- If MRI not available, CT brain and orbits with contrast and CT angiography
- Consider 4-vessel angiography if high clinical suspicion of CCF despite normal CT/MR findings

Treatment

Indirect CCF and asymptomatic:

- Does not need to be treated.
- Monitor for evolution of symptoms.
- Resolve spontaneously in some cases.

Symptomatic/direct CCF:

- Refer to Interventional Radiologists, urgently if necessary for consideration of endovascular treatment
- Glaucoma medication for raised intraocular pressure

- Lubricants/lid taping/moist chamber/temporary tarsorrhaphy for exposure keratopathy
- Bangerter foil/Fresnel prism for symptomatic relief of diplopia

> **GEH Perspectives**
> - *Identifying Symptoms*: When evaluating a patient with severe bilateral conjunctival swelling, be sure to look for signs of optic neuropathy, high intraocular pressure (IOP), and limited ocular motility. These can help distinguish CCF from conjunctivitis.
> - *Conservative Management*: For indirect CCF cases that do not present with optic neuropathy, exposure keratopathy, or high IOP, conservative management may be appropriate, as these cases can often resolve spontaneously.
> - *Need for Early Intervention*: Direct CCF tends to be more symptomatic and typically requires early treatment by interventional radiologists to achieve a good clinical outcome. Prompt referral can make a significant difference in patient care.

Open Access This chapter is licensed under the terms of the Creative Commons Attribution-NonCommercial-NoDerivatives 4.0 International License (http://creativecommons.org/licenses/by-nc-nd/4.0/), which permits any non-commercial use, sharing, distribution and reproduction in any medium or format, as long as you give appropriate credit to the original author(s) and the source, provide a link to the Creative Commons license and indicate if you modified the licensed material. You do not have permission under this license to share adapted material derived from this chapter or parts of it.

The images or other third party material in this chapter are included in the chapter's Creative Commons license, unless indicated otherwise in a credit line to the material. If material is not included in the chapter's Creative Commons license and your intended use is not permitted by statutory regulation or exceeds the permitted use, you will need to obtain permission directly from the copyright holder.

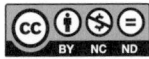

Central Retinal Artery Occlusion (CRAO)

27

Charles Ong and Anna C S Tan

History

- Sudden painless drop in vision
- Vascular risk factors—diabetes, hypertension, dyslipidaemia, and smoking
- If elderly, consider giant cell arteritis (GCA) as an underlying cause
  - Ask for GCA symptoms (temporal headache, scalp tenderness, jaw claudication, polymyalgia rheumatica)

Examination

- Vision loss typically profound—counting fingers or worse
- Presence of RAPD
- Check iris for signs of neovascularisation and consider a gonioscopy to look for neovascularisation in the angles
- Dilated fundus examination looking for signs such as:

C. Ong
Singapore National Eye Centre, Singapore Eye Research Institute, Singapore, Singapore

A. C S Tan (✉)
Department of Medical Retina, Singapore National Eye Centre, Singapore Eye Research Institute, Singapore, Singapore
e-mail: anna.tan.c.s@singhealth.com.sg

© The Author(s) 2026
A. C S Tan et al. (eds.), *The Global Eye Health Handbook*,
https://doi.org/10.1007/978-981-96-8861-6_27

- Retinal pallor
- Cherry red spot
- Retinal emboli
- Assess for underlying cause
  - Carotid bruit, cardiac murmur, irregular pulse suggesting atrial fibrillation
  - Tender nodular pulseless temporal artery suggesting GCA

Investigations

- Widefield colour fundus photo for documentation
- OCT macula to look for inner retinal thinning
- OCTA look for peripheral areas of capillary fall out, NVEs and NVDs, and determine the foveal avascular zone
- Widefield fundus fluorescein angiography especially to look for the presence of vascular diseases in the fellow eye

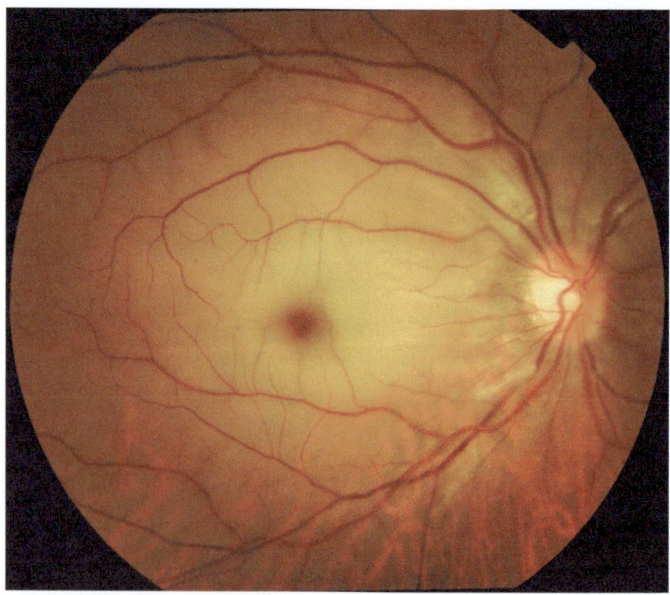

Above fundus photo showing a cherry red spot with a diffusely pale and oedematous retina suggestive of central retinal artery occlusion (CRAO)

Management

- Consider acute ocular resuscitative measures; however, visual prognosis remains guarded
- Principle—induce retinal embolus to dislodge by lowering IOP or with ocular massage and restore retinal perfusion
- Ocular massage
- Intravenous acetazolamide
- Anterior chamber paracentesis
- Topical brimonidine
- Prompt referral to neurology service for stroke workup and management (CRAO is a stroke!)
    - Requires neuroimaging and embolic workup (e.g. carotid ultrasound, echocardiogram, Holter)
- If GCA suspected, perform autoimmune workup and co-manage with physician

> **GEH Perspectives**
> - The prognosis of CRAO is very guarded and complete visual recovery is unlikely.
> - Screening and strict control of cardiovascular risk factors is important to reduce the risk of another CRAO in the fellow eye or subsequent cerebrovascular events.
> - The fellow eye should be assessed and treated for underlying vascular disease and ischaemia as it is the only seeing eye.
> - NVI screening and prompt PRP treatment is important to prevent neovascular glaucoma and the development of a painful blind eye.

Open Access This chapter is licensed under the terms of the Creative Commons Attribution-NonCommercial-NoDerivatives 4.0 International License (http://creativecommons.org/licenses/by-nc-nd/4.0/), which permits any noncommercial use, sharing, distribution and reproduction in any medium or format, as long as you give appropriate credit to the original author(s) and the source, provide a link to the Creative Commons license and indicate if you modified the licensed material. You do not have permission under this license to share adapted material derived from this chapter or parts of it.

The images or other third party material in this chapter are included in the chapter's Creative Commons license, unless indicated otherwise in a credit line to the material. If material is not included in the chapter's Creative Commons license and your intended use is not permitted by statutory regulation or exceeds the permitted use, you will need to obtain permission directly from the copyright holder.

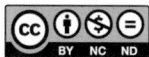

Central Retinal Vein Occlusion

28

Charles Ong and Anna C S Tan

Central/Branch or Hemi-Retinal Vein Occlusion

History

- Drop in vision, metamorphopsia, scotoma, floaters
- Cardiovascular risk factors such as a hypertension, diabetes, hypercholesterolemia, previous history of ischaemic heart disease or stroke
- Modifiable risk factors—smoking, diet, and exercise

Examination

- VA, intraocular pressure, lens status
- Check iris for signs of neovascularisation and consider a gonioscopy to look for neovascularisation in the angles
- Dilated fundus examination looking for signs such as:
  - Flame shaped haemorrhages
  - Tortuous retinal venules

C. Ong
Singapore National Eye Centre, Singapore Eye Research Institute, Singapore, Singapore

A. C S Tan (✉)
Department of Medical Retina, Singapore National Eye Centre, Singapore Eye Research Institute, Singapore, Singapore
e-mail: anna.tan.c.s@singhealth.com.sg

- Cotton wool spots
- Optic disc swelling
- Cystoid macula oedema
- Signs that suggest ischaemic central retinal vein occlusion: poor VA worse than 6/120, RAPD, visual field defect, extensive retinal haemorrhages, and disc swelling

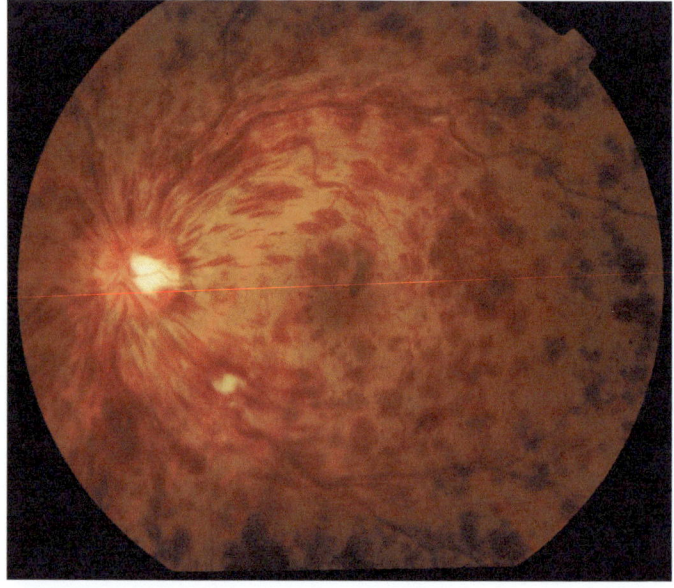

Above fundus photo shows a 'blood and thunder' appearance showing four quadrants of flame shaped haemorrhages, vessel tortuosity, cotton wool spots, and disc swelling suggestive of central retinal vein occlusion (CRVO). The macula appears swollen indicative of cystoid macula oedema (CMO)

Investigations

- Widefield colour fundus photo for documentation
- OCT macula to look for cystoid macula oedema
- OCTA look for peripheral areas of capillary fall out, NVEs and NVDs and determine the foveal avascular zone

- Wide-field fundus fluorescein angiography to be done after haemorrhages resolve to look for >10 disc areas of ischaemia for CRVO, >5 disc diameter for BRVO

Management

- Co-manage with physician for systemic risk factors (diabetes, dyslipidaemia, hypertension)
- Stop smoking
- If young and/or no systemic risk factors, then would suggest further workup by physician for secondary causes (e.g. autoimmune/vasculitic disorders, hypercoagulable states)
- Cystoid macula oedema with vision worse than 6/12—treat with intravitreal anti-VEGF injections
- PRP if neovascularization develops; may consider PRP in select patients (e.g. poor compliance to follow up) if significant ischaemia on FFA but no signs of neovascularisation

GEH Perspectives
- The presence of cotton wool spots and inner retinal thinning seen on the OCT may be signs of an ischaemic fundus and FFA should after haemorrhages clear to determine the extent of capillary fall out.
- Patients should be monitored for a possible ischaemic conversion with increasing signs of haemorrhage and cotton wool spots.
- Macula oedema from RVO requires long-term follow-up and timely IVT for the best visual outcome.
- Patients should be adequately counselled about their disease and should be included in treatment decisions.
- Barriers to long-term treatment and adherence to IVT should be identified and addressed.

Clinic Essentials for Medical Retina Practice
　Slit lamp
　Lenses (e.g. 78D, 90D) for fundus slit lamp indirect ophthalmoscopy
　Optical coherence tomography (OCT) machine
　Intravitreal anti-VEGF injection capabilities
　Retinal lasers
　Ultrasound B scan

Additional Facilities for Medical Retina Practice
　Color and wide field fundus photography
　Fundus autofluorescence
　Fundus fluorescein (FFA) and indocyanine green angiography (ICGA)
　OCT Angiography (OCTA)
　Intravitreal steroid injections

Open Access This chapter is licensed under the terms of the Creative Commons Attribution-NonCommercial-NoDerivatives 4.0 International License (http://creativecommons.org/licenses/by-nc-nd/4.0/), which permits any noncommercial use, sharing, distribution and reproduction in any medium or format, as long as you give appropriate credit to the original author(s) and the source, provide a link to the Creative Commons license and indicate if you modified the licensed material. You do not have permission under this license to share adapted material derived from this chapter or parts of it.

The images or other third party material in this chapter are included in the chapter's Creative Commons license, unless indicated otherwise in a credit line to the material. If material is not included in the chapter's Creative Commons license and your intended use is not permitted by statutory regulation or exceeds the permitted use, you will need to obtain permission directly from the copyright holder.

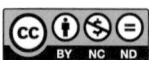

Vitreous Haemorrhage

29

Joshua Lim and Andrew Tsai

Introduction to Surgical Retina

1. Early detection and diagnosis remain important for good outcomes
   (a) It could be helpful to keep in mind that early detection and diagnosis play a key role in achieving better outcomes.
   (b) A comprehensive examination using binocular indirect ophthalmoscopy, with indentation if needed, could be valuable for thorough assessment.
   (c) Clear documentation of the type of retinal detachment, the areas of breaks, and the extent of the detachment, either through photographs or an Amsler-Dubois chart, might also prove useful.
2. Access to diagnostic tools
   (a) Having access to diagnostic tools, like a B scan, especially when the ocular media is hazy, could provide crucial assistance in diagnosis.

J. Lim · A. Tsai (✉)
Singapore National Eye Centre, Singapore Eye Research Institute, Singapore, Singapore
e-mail: andrew.tsai.s.h@singhealth.com.sg

3. Prompt referral to specialists
   (a) Establishing strong referral networks to retinal specialists could help ensure that patients, or those suspected to have a retinal detachment, receive timely treatment.
   (b) Telemedicine might offer further support in facilitating early diagnosis and advice.
4. Surgical skill and upskilling
   (a) It may also be worthwhile to consider making basic retinal detachment surgeries, such as scleral buckling and vitrectomy, more accessible and affordable.
   (b) Investing in training healthcare providers in retinal repair techniques and pre- and post-operative care could go a long way in ensuring that patients receive a good standard of care.
   (c) Collaborating with international organizations and experts might also bring valuable support in advancing surgical techniques and training for local ophthalmologists.
5. Patient education
   (a) Ensuring that patients are aware of the symptoms of retinal detachment, such as photopsia, floaters, and sudden vision changes, and understanding the importance of seeking urgent medical attention, could further help in improving outcomes.

History

- Sudden onset of floaters with progressive blurring of vision
- Ocular trauma
- Ischemic risk factors, especially DM

Examination

- VA
- RAPD
- Raised IOP
- Iris neovascularisation
- Gonioscopy for new vessels at angle
- Fundus examination if possible
- Retinal breaks or detachment
- 3 mirror lens, BIO exam
- Retinal haemorrhages and neovascularisation

Investigations

- Ultrasound B-scan if poor view
- Exclude retinal detachment
- BP and capillary glucose if likely ischemic retinal disease (e.g. DM, retina vein occlusion (RVO), OIS)

Treatment

- Prompt referral to vitreo-retina service if retinal break/retina detachment (RD) is suspected
- If no RAPD or RD present, advise sleeping with head elevation and arrange early review
- Co-management with internist for systemic vascular diseases (Fig. 29.1)

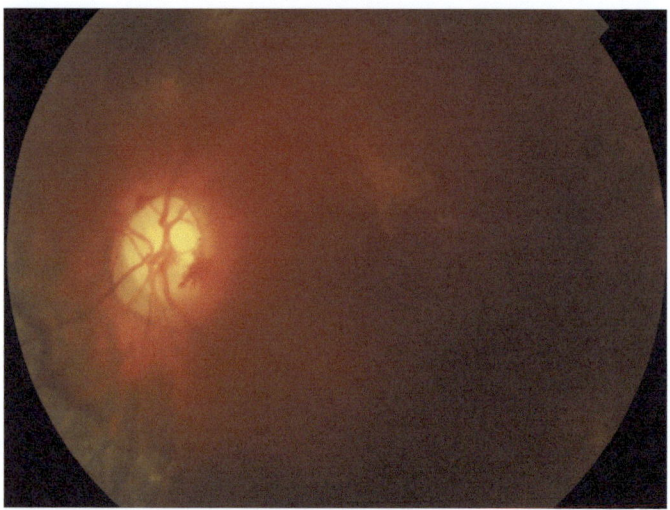

Fig. 29.1 This fundus photo shows diffusely hazy media suggestive of a vitreous haemorrhage (VH), with fronds of new vessels emanating from the disc. There is also some preretinal blood adjacent to the disc. This patient likely has proliferative diabetic retinopathy (PDR) complicated by VH

Clinical Pearls

Common Causes of VH

PDR, RVO, posterior vitreous detachment (PVD), retinal break (most important), RD with VH (most immediately sight threatening), AMD with breakthrough bleed.

About one in ten people with PVD develop a retinal tear, which, if left untreated will develop into a retinal detachment, and a VH increases the risk of RD

GEH Perspectives
- *Return Advice*: Give return advice to patients to return earlier if develop new or worsening symptoms such as flashes of light, curtain like shadow for urgent ocular evaluation.
- *Treat Underlying Aetiology*: Rule out associated retinal tears or detachment through detailed fundus exam. When there is improving fundal view, can carry out laser retinopexy or pan retinal photocoagulation as indicated.
- *Address Underlying Cause*: Encourage adherence to systemic disease control measures such as proper glycaemic control to prevent recurrence.
- *Interim Measures*: In the interim, to advise patients to rest with head elevated to allow blood to settle and improve vision temporarily, avoid strenuous activities that may exacerbate bleeding.

Open Access This chapter is licensed under the terms of the Creative Commons Attribution-NonCommercial-NoDerivatives 4.0 International License (http://creativecommons.org/licenses/by-nc-nd/4.0/), which permits any non-commercial use, sharing, distribution and reproduction in any medium or format, as long as you give appropriate credit to the original author(s) and the source, provide a link to the Creative Commons license and indicate if you modified the licensed material. You do not have permission under this license to share adapted material derived from this chapter or parts of it.

The images or other third party material in this chapter are included in the chapter's Creative Commons license, unless indicated otherwise in a credit line to the material. If material is not included in the chapter's Creative Commons license and your intended use is not permitted by statutory regulation or exceeds the permitted use, you will need to obtain permission directly from the copyright holder.

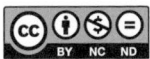

# Retinal Detachment

Joshua Lim, Andrew Tsai, and Ian Yeo

History

- Sudden onset of floaters and flashes
- Progressive visual field loss, may experience a curtain effect—ascertain duration of RD and duration of macula-off (when did the central vision get affected)
- Myopia
- Recent intraocular surgery, IVT, or laser procedures
- Family history of RD and relevant underlying systemic diseases (e.g. Marfan, Stickler)
- Ocular trauma

Examination

- VA and RAPD
- IOP
- Lens status
- Vitreous pigment (Schaffer sign) or haemorrhage
- Retinal breaks and detachment (macula on/off)
- Illustrate RD findings properly—can use Amsler-Dubois charting

J. Lim · A. Tsai (✉) · I. Yeo
Singapore National Eye Centre, Singapore Eye Research Institute, Singapore, Singapore
e-mail: andrew.tsai.s.h@singhealth.com.sg

Investigations

- Ultrasound B-scan if no view of retina
- Preoperative workup
- Keep patient fasted until vitreo-retina fellow gives
- Instructions

Treatment

- Prompt referral to vitreo-retina service, especially if macula-on RD
- Rest in bed, posture depending on RD configuration
- Prepare for operation (Fig. 30.1)

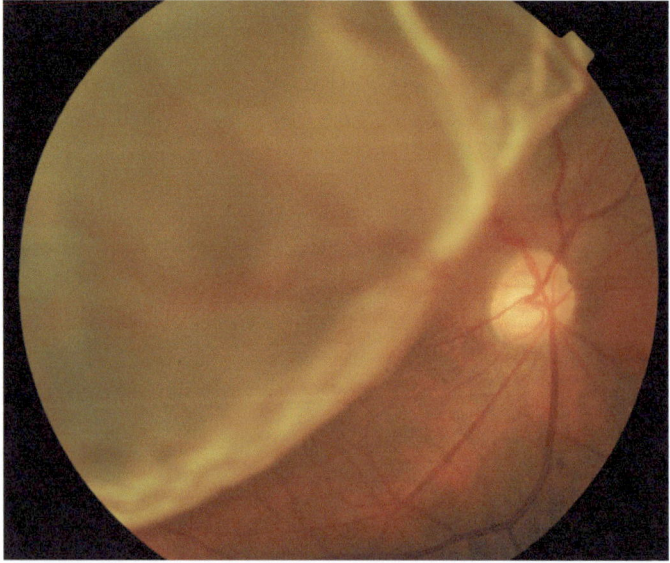

Fig. 30.1 This fundus photo shows a bullous macula-off superior rhegmatogenous retinal detachment (RRD) extending from 7 o'clock to 1 o'clock. The peripheries will need to be examined to locate the break

> **GEH Perspectives**
> - *Follow Lincoff's Rules*: When assessing a patient with retinal detachment, remember Lincoff's rules to determine the best management approach. This structured approach can help guide your decision-making for optimal outcomes.
> - *Consider Scleral Buckling*: Always ask yourself if the RD can be treated effectively with scleral buckling alone. This less invasive option can be beneficial for certain types of detachments and may lead to quicker recovery for the patient.
> - *Advise on Gas Management*: If gas is used in the treatment, educate patients on proper positioning to maintain the gas bubble's effectiveness. Additionally, provide clear guidance on air travel restrictions to prevent complications—it is important for patients to understand how to care for their eyes during recovery!

Open Access This chapter is licensed under the terms of the Creative Commons Attribution-NonCommercial-NoDerivatives 4.0 International License (http://creativecommons.org/licenses/by-nc-nd/4.0/), which permits any non-commercial use, sharing, distribution and reproduction in any medium or format, as long as you give appropriate credit to the original author(s) and the source, provide a link to the Creative Commons license and indicate if you modified the licensed material. You do not have permission under this license to share adapted material derived from this chapter or parts of it.

The images or other third party material in this chapter are included in the chapter's Creative Commons license, unless indicated otherwise in a credit line to the material. If material is not included in the chapter's Creative Commons license and your intended use is not permitted by statutory regulation or exceeds the permitted use, you will need to obtain permission directly from the copyright holder.

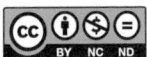

Infections: Exogenous (Post-operative) Endophthalmitis

31

Joshua Lim and Andrew Tsai

History

- Date of surgery and complications (especially posterior capsular rupture)
- Pain, redness, and swelling
- Blurring of vision
- Systemic conditions, e.g. diabetes mellitus

Examination

- VA (better or worse than light perception) and RAPD
- Anterior segment
- Blepharitis and eyelid swelling
- Conjunctival injection and chemosis
- Corneal oedema, abscesses (especially at sutures and bleb), wound leaks
- Intraocular pressure
- Anterior chamber cells, flare, fibrin, and hypopyon
- Posterior segment

J. Lim · A. Tsai (✉)
Singapore National Eye Centre, Singapore Eye Research Institute, Singapore, Singapore
e-mail: andrew.tsai.s.h@singhealth.com.sg

- Vitritis
- Retinal haemorrhages and vasculitis
- Disc hyperaemia and swelling
- Ultrasound B-scan if no view

Investigations

- Ultrasound B-scan if retina not visible to exclude vitritis
- Full blood count, C-reactive protein

Vitreous Tap

- Vitreous tap with 23-gauge needle (guarded at 10 mm) on 5 mL syringe
- Enter vitreous cavity through pars plana 3.5 mm (if pseudophakic; 4 mm if phakic) posterior to limbus, aiming to centre of globe
- Aspirate 0.2 mL of vitreous—send for gram stain and cultures
- For non-yielding/dry taps, repeat with larger needle or consider trying a different site

Treatment

- Post-operative endophthalmitis is an ocular emergency, and treatment must commence urgently
- Consider early vitrectomy
- Admit
- Refer to an Infectious Diseases team

If Visual Acuity Is Light Perception or Worse

- *Keep patient fasted, prepare for vitrectomy*
- *Inform vitreo-retina fellow promptly*

- Intravitreal antibiotic: Vancomycin 1 mg in 0.1 mL and ceftazidime 2.25 mg in 0.1 mL
- Injected separately via pars plana with 27-gauge needle and 1 mL syringes

Medications

- *Topical cefazolin and gentamicin every hourly*
- *Oral ciprofloxacin 500 mg twice a day*
- *Cycloplegia*
- *± Glaucoma medication*
- *Oral analgesia*
- Inform guarded visual prognosis
- Inform primary surgeon/infection control committee

Differential Diagnosis

- *Toxic Anterior Segment Syndrome (onset 24 hours after cataract surgery* versus *exogenous endophthalmitis 3–7 days after cataract surgery)*

Open Access This chapter is licensed under the terms of the Creative Commons Attribution-NonCommercial-NoDerivatives 4.0 International License (http://creativecommons.org/licenses/by-nc-nd/4.0/), which permits any non-commercial use, sharing, distribution and reproduction in any medium or format, as long as you give appropriate credit to the original author(s) and the source, provide a link to the Creative Commons license and indicate if you modified the licensed material. You do not have permission under this license to share adapted material derived from this chapter or parts of it.

The images or other third party material in this chapter are included in the chapter's Creative Commons license, unless indicated otherwise in a credit line to the material. If material is not included in the chapter's Creative Commons license and your intended use is not permitted by statutory regulation or exceeds the permitted use, you will need to obtain permission directly from the copyright holder.

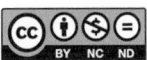

Infections: IVT-Related Endophthalmitis

Joshua Lim and Andrew Tsai

History

- Date of last intravitreal injection, indication, and agent used
- Pain, redness
- Blurring of vision

Examination

- VA
- IOP
- RAPD
- AC cells, flare, hypopyon, fibrin
- Vitritis, retinitis, retinal haemorrhages

Investigations

- B-scan if no view of posterior segment
- Vitreous tap (as above)

J. Lim · A. Tsai (✉)
Singapore National Eye Centre, Singapore Eye Research Institute, Singapore, Singapore
e-mail: andrew.tsai.s.h@singhealth.com.sg

Treatment

- Admit patient
- Vitreous tap and IVT antibiotics
- Keep patient fasted, keep in view for vitrectomy
- Topical antibiotics
- Atropine 1% three times a day
- Consider oral ciprofloxacin or moxifloxacin
- Consider early vitrectomy
- Trace Gram stain after 1–2 h, and cultures after 24 h

GEH Perspectives—Post-Operative and Intravitreal-Related Endophthalmitis
- *IVT-related endophthalmitis represents a sentinel event that requires adequate investigation to reduce the risk of infection to other patients treated during the same period.*
  1. Early detection and prompt treatment is key
     (a) Patients should ideally get close post-operative monitoring.
     (b) Education of patients on key symptoms of endophthalmitis (e.g. redness, pain, blurring of vision) and encourage them to surface issues immediately.
     (c) Rapid response: Immediate treatment is critical. Initiate broad spectrum antibiotics as soon as endophthalmitis is suspected.
     (d) Know what are the common pathogens that may afflict the region you are working in.
  2. Aseptic surgical techniques for primary prevention
     (a) Maintenance of a sterile environment before and during surgery is most important.
     (b) Administer prophylactic antibiotics, especially following surgery.
  3. Resource utilisation and training
     (a) Understand the common pathogens in the region, develop and adhere to guidelines if available for empirical treatment.

(b) Capacity building—training healthcare workers on the identification and management of endophthalmitis at a primary care setting can bring better outcomes to patients.
4. Expedient referral systems
   (a) Establish a robust referral system to ensure patients are quickly referred to higher level facilities when specialist care is available.
   (b) Utilise telemedicine if resources are spread across a large geographical area to bridge access to remote sites.
5. Reliable documentation and reporting
   (a) Maintain detailed records of surgical notes, intra-operative complications, pre- and post-operative prescriptions.
   (b) Maintain detailed clerking records of patient's progress and outcomes.

Frequently audit data to improve local practices and outcomes.

Open Access This chapter is licensed under the terms of the Creative Commons Attribution-NonCommercial-NoDerivatives 4.0 International License (http://creativecommons.org/licenses/by-nc-nd/4.0/), which permits any non-commercial use, sharing, distribution and reproduction in any medium or format, as long as you give appropriate credit to the original author(s) and the source, provide a link to the Creative Commons license and indicate if you modified the licensed material. You do not have permission under this license to share adapted material derived from this chapter or parts of it.

The images or other third party material in this chapter are included in the chapter's Creative Commons license, unless indicated otherwise in a credit line to the material. If material is not included in the chapter's Creative Commons license and your intended use is not permitted by statutory regulation or exceeds the permitted use, you will need to obtain permission directly from the copyright holder.

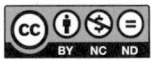

Neuro-Ophthalmology: Optic Neuritis

33

Reuben Foo, Shweta Singhal, and Umapathi Thirugnanam

Introduction to Neuro-Ophthalmology

Clinical Essentials

Most neuro-ophthalmological conditions are diagnosed on history and examination.

Always ask for red flags (Raised intracranial pressure symptoms/previous cancer history).

Optic nerve function assessment includes visual acuity (near and distance), confrontation fields, colour vision and pupil examination.

Cover test and alternate cover test in different directions of gaze will diagnose most ocular motor pathologies.

Examine contiguous cranial nerve V1,2,3 VII and VIII to help localise site of intracranial pathology.

Refer urgently for neuroimaging when suspecting intracranial pathology.

Equipment that would help:

Apps on mobile phones can be used to check VA and colour vision in remote settings.

R. Foo · S. Singhal (✉) · U. Thirugnanam
Singapore National Eye Centre, Singapore Eye Research Institute, Singapore, Singapore
e-mail: shweta.singhal@singhealth.com.sg

A pointed and focused source of light (direct ophthalmoscope or muscle light) gives best results for pupil examination.

Red targets (red capped eye drop bottle) can be used to pick up subtle visual field defects/chart central scotomas in the absence of formal perimetry.

HVF and OCT RNFL GCIPL measurements are helpful accessory tests when available.

Optic Neuritis History

- Visual loss over hours to days
- Pain with eye movement, may precede visual symptoms
- Recent febrile illness
- History of other neurological symptoms (focal neurological deficits)

Examination

- Reduced VA, severe disproportionate drop in colour vision
- Visual field defects/central scotomas on confrontation testing
- Significant RAPD despite good VA
- Fundoscopy may show normal disc, slight hyperaemia, or significant disc swelling
- In cases where disc appearance is normal, look for subtle retinal pathology

Investigations

- Confirm optic neuritis by looking for contrast enhancement of the optic nerve/chiasm on MRI anterior visual pathway and brain (also detects white matter plaques in case of MS)

- If optic neuritis is confirmed,
  - Pre-steroid work-up
  - NMO (Neuromyelitis optica) and MOG (Myelin oligodendrocyte glycoprotein antibody testing) (PRIOR to starting steroids)
- In cases where MRI is inconclusive/NMO and MOG antibody testing is negative, and patient doesn't respond to steroids, expand workup as follows:
  - Autoimmune screen: Anti-nuclear antibodies (ANA), Anti-double stranded DNA (dsDNA), Antineutrophil cytoplasmic antibody indirect immunofluorescence (ANCA IIF), Anti-myeloperoxidase (MPO), Anti proteinase 3 (PR3), Extractable nuclear antigen (ENA) screen & ENA profile, Rheumatoid factor (RF), Lupus anticoagulant, Anticardiolipin Immunoglobulin M (IgM) & IgG
  - Refer Neurology
  - Lumbar puncture for cerebrospinal fluid (CSF) analysis
  - MRI Spine

Treatment

- Once diagnosis is confirmed, the first line of treatment is with intravenous (IV) methylprednisolone (3–5 days/1 g per day).
- If no response, consider plasmapheresis/intravenous immunoglobulins.
- Manage with neuro-ophthalmology/neurology

GEH Perspectives
- *Know the Common Causes*: When evaluating a patient with optic neuritis, remember that multiple sclerosis (MS), neuromyelitis optica (NMO), and myelin oligodendrocyte glycoprotein (MOG)-related optic neuritis are the most common causes. Keeping these in mind can guide your approach to diagnosis and treatment.
- *Act Quickly*: The key to effective treatment is confirming the diagnosis with appropriate neuroimaging as soon as possible. Early initiation of intravenous steroids can make a significant difference in patient outcomes.
- *Consider Other Factors*: If tests come back negative for the usual suspects, don't forget to consider autoimmune, infectious, or para-infectious causes. A comprehensive approach can help ensure no underlying condition is overlooked.

Open Access This chapter is licensed under the terms of the Creative Commons Attribution-NonCommercial-NoDerivatives 4.0 International License (http://creativecommons.org/licenses/by-nc-nd/4.0/), which permits any noncommercial use, sharing, distribution and reproduction in any medium or format, as long as you give appropriate credit to the original author(s) and the source, provide a link to the Creative Commons license and indicate if you modified the licensed material. You do not have permission under this license to share adapted material derived from this chapter or parts of it.

The images or other third party material in this chapter are included in the chapter's Creative Commons license, unless indicated otherwise in a credit line to the material. If material is not included in the chapter's Creative Commons license and your intended use is not permitted by statutory regulation or exceeds the permitted use, you will need to obtain permission directly from the copyright holder.

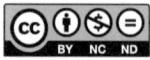

# Neuro-Ophthalmology: Anterior Ischemic Optic Neuropathy (AION)— Arteritic and Non-arteritic

Reuben Foo, Shweta Singhal, and Umapathi Thirugnanam

History

Non-arteritic

- Acute unilateral painless sudden onset visual loss, often on awakening
- Altitudinal field loss (superior or inferior half of field)
- Risk factors: Vascular risk factors (diabetes/hypertension/hyperlipidaemia/smoking/obstructive sleep apnoea)—snoring or daytime somnolence, and phosphodiesterase (PDE) inhibitors (for males)

Arteritic

- Acute, painful visual loss
- Can have episodes of transient visual loss

Symptoms of giant cell arteritis (GCA)

- Localised headache
- Fever, malaise, weight loss
- Jaw claudication, scalp tenderness
- Proximal myalgia and arthralgia

Examination

Non-arteritic:

- In acute cases, affected disc is swollen and hyperaemic (+/− disc peripapillary splinter haemorrhages) (Fig. 34.1).
- Disc swelling is usually worse superiorly or inferiorly and corresponds inversely with area of visual field loss.

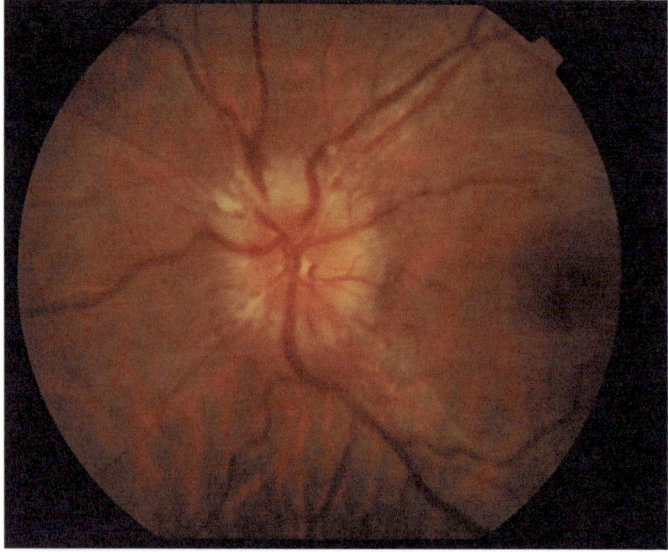

Fig. 34.1 This disc photo shows a diffusely hyperaemic swollen disc with peripapillary splinter haemorrhages in a disc-at-risk. The margins are elevated with obscuration of the vessels

- Unaffected disc will be a small crowded disc with small cup disc ratio (disc at risk).

Arteritic:

- Chalky white, pallid disc swelling, signs of central retinal artery occlusion (see Chap. 28)
- Contiguous cranial nerves (CN3, 4, 5, 6)
- Proptosis
- Palpate temporal artery for pulses and tender nodular cord like swelling of temporal artery

Investigations

Non-arteritic

- Blood pressure (BP), capillary glucose, fasting lipids

Arteritic

- Full blood count (FBC) (increased platelets), Erythrocyte Sedimentation Rate (ESR), C-reactive protein (CRP)
- Pre-steroid workup (e.g. if suspecting GCA)
- Urgent temporal artery biopsy
- Ultrasound of temporal artery (characteristic dark wall swelling [halo] and acute occlusions)

Others

- Additional workup for young patients or no vascular risk factors
- ANA, anti-dsDNA, RF, anti-phospholipid, ENA profile
- Homocysteine

Treatment

Non-arteritic

- Control underlying systemic vascular risk factors for non-arteritic AION
- Can consider starting brimonidine tartrate (neuroprotective) to affected eye

Arteritic

- Suspect GCA in cases of elevated ESR/CRP, arrange urgent temporal artery biopsy.
- Co-manage with rheumatology, consider IV methylprednisolone in consultation with Neuro-ophthalmology and Oculoplastic service.
- Suspect rarer causes of AION (e.g. Takayasu arteritis, polyarteritis nodosa, relapsing polychondritis) in young patients or atypical presentations

---

GEH Perspectives
- *Recognize the Signs*: NAION often presents as a common cause of a sudden, painless loss of vision in one eye. Be on the lookout for altitudinal disc swelling and corresponding visual field loss. It's essential to assess for significant vascular risk factors in your patients.
- *Optimize Vascular Health*: While there's no specific treatment for NAION, managing the patient's vascular risk factors is crucial. Discuss lifestyle changes and medications that can help improve their overall vascular health and provide counseling about visual prognosis, including the risks to the opposite eye if these factors aren't addressed.

- *Don't Overlook GCA*: Giant Cell Arteritis (GCA) is less common but can be life-threatening and vision-threatening. For patients over 50 presenting with severe vision loss, headache, and a pale swollen disc, it's vital to suspect GCA. Prompt steroid therapy is essential to preserve both sight and life. Make sure to refer these patients to an internist or rheumatologist if available for comprehensive management.

Open Access This chapter is licensed under the terms of the Creative Commons Attribution-NonCommercial-NoDerivatives 4.0 International License (http://creativecommons.org/licenses/by-nc-nd/4.0/), which permits any non-commercial use, sharing, distribution and reproduction in any medium or format, as long as you give appropriate credit to the original author(s) and the source, provide a link to the Creative Commons license and indicate if you modified the licensed material. You do not have permission under this license to share adapted material derived from this chapter or parts of it.

The images or other third party material in this chapter are included in the chapter's Creative Commons license, unless indicated otherwise in a credit line to the material. If material is not included in the chapter's Creative Commons license and your intended use is not permitted by statutory regulation or exceeds the permitted use, you will need to obtain permission directly from the copyright holder.

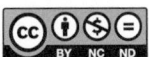

Neuro-Ophthalmology: Unilateral Disc Swelling

Reuben Foo, Shweta Singhal, and Umapathi Thirugnanam

History

- Symptoms: BOV, vision being blocked by a patch (scotoma)
- Symptoms of raised ICP—headache, nausea, vomiting, pulsatile tinnitus, transient obscuration of vision, and diplopia
- Symptom onset, duration, and progression

If suspecting inflammatory optic neuritis such as with multiple sclerosis, NMO spectrum disease, MOG-related disease, also ask for:

- Previous episodes
- Pain on EOM, retro orbital ache
- Upper limb/lower limb weakness
- Vomiting/Bowel/urinary incontinence

Other relevant history:

- Autoimmune
- Recent infections or immunisation (vaccination-induced)

- Trauma
- Previous malignancy or radiation (compressive/radiation-induced)
- Vascular risk factors (NAAION)
- Scalp tenderness, jaw claudication (AAION)
- Pain (posterior scleritis/uveitis)

Examination

- Optic nerve function, including colour vision (colour vision loss disproportionate to visual acuity loss in optic neuritis)
- Contiguous cranial nerves, including ocular motility and corneo facial sensation (exclude orbital mass restriction and orbital apex syndrome)
- Look for proptosis with Hertel's exophthalmometer
- Establish nature of disc swelling—swelling vs hyperaemia, blurred disc margins, peripapillary haemorrhages, spontaneous venous pulsation, Paton's line, obscuration of vessels, optociliary shunt (chronicity)
- Look for associated ocular pathology with a dilated fundal exam: retinitis/vitritis, central retinal vein occlusion, central retinal artery occlusion (GCA), choroidal folds, diabetic retinopathy (papillitis), neuroretinitis, posterior uveitis

Investigations

- Formal visual fields to establish nature of visual field defect which helps with DDx (e.g. central scotoma in optic neuritis vs altitudinal defect in NA AION)
- Structural imaging of optic nerve, e.g. optical coherence tomography of optic nerve fibre layer (to confirm disc swelling and to monitor disease progression)
- FBC ESR CRP, vascular risk factors
- Infective, autoimmune, and pre-steroid workup
- Consider MOG and NMO antibodies if high suspicion

- MRI brain with contrast ± spinal cord (transverse myelitis—lesion extending continuously over ≥3 vertebral segments)
- Ultrasound B-scan for posterior scleritis and optic disc drusen

Management

Treat underlying cause

Open Access This chapter is licensed under the terms of the Creative Commons Attribution-NonCommercial-NoDerivatives 4.0 International License (http://creativecommons.org/licenses/by-nc-nd/4.0/), which permits any noncommercial use, sharing, distribution and reproduction in any medium or format, as long as you give appropriate credit to the original author(s) and the source, provide a link to the Creative Commons license and indicate if you modified the licensed material. You do not have permission under this license to share adapted material derived from this chapter or parts of it.

The images or other third party material in this chapter are included in the chapter's Creative Commons license, unless indicated otherwise in a credit line to the material. If material is not included in the chapter's Creative Commons license and your intended use is not permitted by statutory regulation or exceeds the permitted use, you will need to obtain permission directly from the copyright holder.

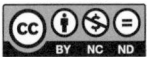

Neuro-Ophthalmology: Bilateral Disc Swelling

36

Reuben Foo, Shweta Singhal, and Umapathi Thirugnanam

History

- Symptoms: BOV, visual field disturbance
- Symptoms of raised intracranial pressure—posture-dependent headache/worse on coughing/straining/Valsalva, nausea, vomiting, pulsatile tinnitus, transient obscuration of vision, diplopia
- Symptom onset, duration, and progression
- Focal neurological deficits (numbness/weakness)
- Vascular risk factors—hypertension (malignant HTN)
- Neck stiffness, fever, photophobia (meningitis)
- Pain (posterior scleritis/uveitis)
- Pain on eye movement/Uthoff phenomenon (inflammatory optic neuritis)
- Recent infection or vaccination (consecutive optic neuritis)
- Cancer, hypercoagulable state, oral contraceptives (Venous sinus thrombosis)
- Medication use—tetracycline, vitamin A/retinoids, NSAID, cyclosporine, oral contraceptives (dural venous thrombosis/idiopathic intracranial hypertension), steroids, lithium withdrawal

---

R. Foo · S. Singhal (✉) · U. Thirugnanam
Singapore National Eye Centre, Singapore Eye Research Institute, Singapore, Singapore
e-mail: shweta.singhal@singhealth.com.sg

Examination

- Potentially life-threatening emergency
- Check BP and temperature; ensure haemodynamically stable
- Assess for features of meningitis like fever and neck stiffness
- Optic nerve function—usually good in papilledema except visual field—enlarged blind spot/peripheral field constriction
- Contiguous cranial nerves, including eye movements (false localising sign of cranial nerve six palsy), corneal/facial sensation
- Cover/alternate cover tests (in primary, left, and right gaze for esotropia)
- IOP, anterior segment examination: uveitis/scleritis
- Visualisation of optic nerve swelling, spontaneous venous pulsation (Fig. 36.1)
- Dilated fundus exam: CRVO, diabetic retinopathy, uveitis

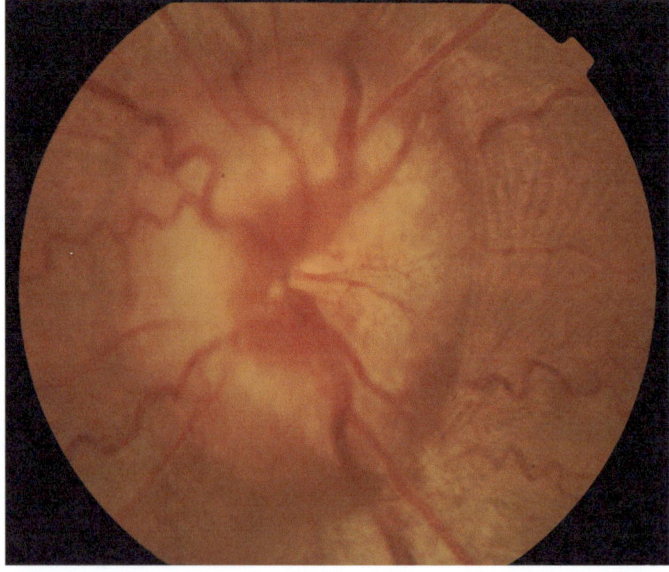

Fig. 36.1 This photo shows a diffusely swollen and hyperaemic disc with obscuration of the disc margins and peripapillary vessels. There are tortuous vessels around the disc and Paton's lines temporally as well

Investigations

- Neuroimaging—MRI brain (looking for tumour, hydrocephalus, meningeal lesion) and orbits with contrast and MRV to exclude space-occupying lesions and cerebral/dural venous sinus thrombosis, white matter lesions
- CT brain to exclude blood if emergent
- Keep in view prompt referral to a neurologist for co-management and lumbar puncture to look for raised ICP and CSF composition to rule out a meningeal process
- *Raised opening pressure—>25 cm H_2O* in lateral decubitus position
- CSF composition for meningitis: glucose (low), protein, gram stain, syphilis, TB PCR, cultures
- FBC, ESR, CRP, renal panel
- Formal visual field perimetry
- Endocrine evaluation for Cushing's, Addison's, thyroid
- +/− Autoimmune screen, microbiological: infective screen, pre-steroid workup, anti-MOG, anti-NMO antibody

Management

- Comanage with neurology
- Urgent referral to internist for malignant HTN
- Treat underlying cause
- Stop reversible causes, e.g. medications

Idiopathic Intracranial Hypertension

Treat Secondary Causes
- Stop drugs
- Systemic disease by co-managing with internist (Cushing's, Addison's disease)
- Refer to sleep clinic for Obstructive Sleep Apnoea (OSA)

- Refer to the weight management clinic. Weight loss reduction of 10% from baseline, sodium reduction
- Monitor optic nerve function serially

Medical Treatment—If Optic Neuropathy or Symptomatic Raised ICP
- Oral acetazolamide if no contraindications
- Or frusemide or topiramate (inhibits carbonic anhydrase—good for headaches, helps weight loss, but more side effects)
- Serial monitoring with visual fields

Surgical
- *Intractable headache*: Neurosurgery management for CSF diversion procedures—ventriculoperitoneal (VP) shunt or lumboperitoneal (LP) shunt despite maximally tolerated medical therapy
- *Worsening VF*: Optic nerve sheath fenestration (ONSF) only if ON function severely compressed despite maximally tolerated medical therapy
- If not fit for the above, e.g. pregnant ladies (cannot take acetazolamide or topiramate) then therapeutic LPs (however, CSF usually replenishes in 1–2 h)

GEH Perspectives
- *Act Swiftly with Bilateral Disc Swelling*: If you observe bilateral disc swelling, treat it as a potentially life-threatening condition until proven otherwise. Prompt action is crucial, so manage it as an emergency.
- *Initial Assessments Matter*: Start by checking the patient's blood pressure and temperature to rule out malignant hypertension and meningitis. These initial assessments can provide valuable insights into the underlying cause.
- *Utilize Neuroimaging*: When neuroimaging is available, opt for a contrast-enhanced MRI of the brain and orbits, along with an MR venogram. This can help identify

potential causes such as intracranial tumors, optic neuritis, or venous sinus thrombosis.
- *Don't Skip Lumbar Puncture Protocols*: If a lumbar puncture is necessary, always check the opening pressure to diagnose raised intracranial pressure accurately. Remember, CSF pressure can be elevated even if the MRI scan appears normal, so this step is vital.
- *Address Underlying Factors in IIH*: When treating Idiopathic Intracranial Hypertension (IIH), focus on identifying and addressing any underlying risk factors. This approach is essential for preventing recurrences and may reduce the need for long-term medical or surgical interventions

Open Access This chapter is licensed under the terms of the Creative Commons Attribution-NonCommercial-NoDerivatives 4.0 International License (http://creativecommons.org/licenses/by-nc-nd/4.0/), which permits any noncommercial use, sharing, distribution and reproduction in any medium or format, as long as you give appropriate credit to the original author(s) and the source, provide a link to the Creative Commons license and indicate if you modified the licensed material. You do not have permission under this license to share adapted material derived from this chapter or parts of it.

The images or other third party material in this chapter are included in the chapter's Creative Commons license, unless indicated otherwise in a credit line to the material. If material is not included in the chapter's Creative Commons license and your intended use is not permitted by statutory regulation or exceeds the permitted use, you will need to obtain permission directly from the copyright holder.

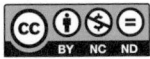

Diplopia: Oculomotor Palsy (CN3)

Reuben Foo, Shweta Singhal, and Umapathi Thirugnanam

History

- Droopy lids
- Binocular double vision
- Pain, headache, vomiting
- Rapid vs. gradual onset of symptoms
- Vascular risk factors (DM, HTN, HLD, IHD)
- Previous history of malignancy

Examination

- Large nonreactive pupil on the affected side with anisocoria worse in the light
- Ptosis, complete or incomplete
- Extraocular motility limitation—eye may be in a 'down and out' position if complete limitation
- Determine if isolated or involving other cranial nerves
- Determine if limitation complete or incomplete

- Look for signs of aberrant regeneration
- Focal neurological deficits (e.g. hemiparesis, hemianesthesia)
- Proptosis

Investigations

Pupil-Involved or Incomplete Third Nerve Palsy

- Life-threatening emergency
- Admit and obtain urgent MRI brain and orbits, MRA angiogram to exclude aneurysm or tumour (consider CT angiogram in the emergency setting)
- Monitor for pupil involvement if not already involved

Pupil Not Involved and Complete Third Nerve Palsy

- BP and capillary glucose: Manage vascular risk factors

> **GEH Perspectives**
> - *Always Consider Aneurysms*: When you encounter patients with pupil-involving third nerve palsies, keep in mind that a posterior communicating artery aneurysm is the likely cause until proven otherwise. This awareness is crucial for timely intervention.
> - *Watch for Subtle Signs*: Be vigilant with patients showing a history of slowly worsening ptosis, even if their third nerve palsy is incomplete and does not involve the pupil. This could indicate a mass lesion that is gradually expanding, and early identification is key to effective management.

Open Access This chapter is licensed under the terms of the Creative Commons Attribution-NonCommercial-NoDerivatives 4.0 International License (http://creativecommons.org/licenses/by-nc-nd/4.0/), which permits any non-commercial use, sharing, distribution and reproduction in any medium or format, as long as you give appropriate credit to the original author(s) and the source, provide a link to the Creative Commons license and indicate if you modified the licensed material. You do not have permission under this license to share adapted material derived from this chapter or parts of it.

The images or other third party material in this chapter are included in the chapter's Creative Commons license, unless indicated otherwise in a credit line to the material. If material is not included in the chapter's Creative Commons license and your intended use is not permitted by statutory regulation or exceeds the permitted use, you will need to obtain permission directly from the copyright holder.

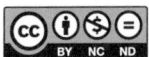

Diplopia: Trochlear Palsy (CN4)

Reuben Foo, Shweta Singhal, and Umapathi Thirugnanam

History

- Vertical diplopia, especially when reading or walking (looking down)
- Establish if onset is acute or gradual intermittent (ischemic/traumatic palsy vs decompensated congenital CN IV palsy)
- Ask for raised ICP symptoms
- Head trauma, especially high-velocity closed head injuries
- Vascular risk factors (e.g. DM, HTN, HLD, IHD)
- Old photos to look for a previously developed abnormal head posture which may suggest chronicity

Examination

- Affected eye will be hypertrophic.
- On cover/alternate cover test, hypertropia will be worse on opposite gaze and ipsilateral head tilt.
- Abnormal head posture (tilted away from hypertropic eye).

R. Foo · S. Singhal (✉) · U. Thirugnanam
Singapore National Eye Centre, Singapore Eye Research Institute, Singapore, Singapore
e-mail: shweta.singhal@singhealth.com.sg

- Facial asymmetry suggesting long-standing or congenital fourth nerve palsy.
- Examine contiguous cranial nerves to see if palsy is isolated.

Investigations

- Urgent neuroimaging (MRI brain with orbits contrasted) if multiple cranial nerves are involved, the onset is gradual and progressive, or the patient had head trauma
- Check BP, fasting blood sugar, and lipids

Treatment

- Manage underlying cause
- If no red flags and acute onset in a patient with vascular risk factors, can be monitored for improvement over 4–6 weeks
- If no signs of improvement after 1 month, consider neuroimaging
- Fresnel prism or Bangerter foil for symptomatic diplopia

> **GEH Perspectives**
>
> *Monitor Acute Onset*: In patients with vascular risk factors who present with acute onset of CN IV palsies, and without symptoms of raised intracranial pressure, prior trauma, or a history of malignancy, consider monitoring them closely. You can provide symptomatic treatment for diplopia over a 4–6 week period to see if symptoms improve.
>
> *Seek Imaging if No Improvement*: If there's no improvement after the monitoring period, it's a good idea to proceed with neuroimaging to rule out any underlying issues.
>
> *Assess for Chronicity*: For patients with a non-acute onset, look for old photographs that might show abnormal head posture or an increased prism fusion range. These clues can help you determine the chronicity of the condition and guide your management approach.

Open Access This chapter is licensed under the terms of the Creative Commons Attribution-NonCommercial-NoDerivatives 4.0 International License (http://creativecommons.org/licenses/by-nc-nd/4.0/), which permits any noncommercial use, sharing, distribution and reproduction in any medium or format, as long as you give appropriate credit to the original author(s) and the source, provide a link to the Creative Commons license and indicate if you modified the licensed material. You do not have permission under this license to share adapted material derived from this chapter or parts of it.

The images or other third party material in this chapter are included in the chapter's Creative Commons license, unless indicated otherwise in a credit line to the material. If material is not included in the chapter's Creative Commons license and your intended use is not permitted by statutory regulation or exceeds the permitted use, you will need to obtain permission directly from the copyright holder.

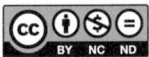

Diplopia: Abducens Nerve Palsy (CN6)

Reuben Foo, Shweta Singhal, and Umapathi Thirugnanam

History

- Horizontal diplopia, worse for distance and better for near
- Headache, nausea, and vomiting
- Transient visual obscuration
- Head trauma
- Nasopharyngeal carcinoma (NPC) or radiotherapy to head
- Vascular risk factors

Examination

- Abduction deficits, unilateral or bilateral
- Esotropia on cover testing
- Involvement of contiguous cranial nerves (III/IV/V/VII, VIII)
- Papilledema (false localising sixth nerve palsy)
- Proptosis

R. Foo · S. Singhal (✉) · U. Thirugnanam
Singapore National Eye Centre, Singapore Eye Research Institute, Singapore, Singapore
e-mail: shweta.singhal@singhealth.com.sg

Investigations

- BP and capillary glucose (non-urgent fasting glucose and lipids)

  Urgent neuroimaging is required in certain cases, for instance:

- Gradual onset progressive binocular double vision
- Bilateral sixth nerve palsy
- Papilledema, suspicion of raised ICP
- Multiple cranial nerve palsies

Treatment

- Prompt referral to neurosurgery if evidence of raised ICP or space-occupying lesion is present.
- Refer to otolaryngology to exclude NPC.
- Manage vascular risk factors.
- Fresnel prism or Bangerter foil for symptomatic diplopia.

GEH Perspectives
- Any CN6 palsy that is not isolated must be evaluated with neuroimaging. This includes even minor symptoms like facial pain/ blocked ears etc.
- Nasoendoscopic evaluation of patients with CN6 palsies is important to rule out nasopharyngeal cancer which is a common life threatening cause of CN6 palsies particularly in endemic regions.

Multiple cranial nerve dictum:

- *All cranial nerves except 1 and 2 arise from the brainstem, so exclude brainstem lesions*
- *All cranial nerves traverse the meninges, so exclude meningitis*

- *Cranial nerves are grouped* e.g. *cerebellopontine angle, cavernous sinus, orbital apex*
- *Myasthenia gravis and Guillain-Barré can mimic multiple cranial nerve palsies*
- *Diabetics typically only suffer one cranial nerve palsy at a time, so exclude other causes for multiple cranial nerve palsies in a diabetic patient*

Consider raised intracranial pressure as a cause of false localising CN6 palsy

Open Access This chapter is licensed under the terms of the Creative Commons Attribution-NonCommercial-NoDerivatives 4.0 International License (http://creativecommons.org/licenses/by-nc-nd/4.0/), which permits any non-commercial use, sharing, distribution and reproduction in any medium or format, as long as you give appropriate credit to the original author(s) and the source, provide a link to the Creative Commons license and indicate if you modified the licensed material. You do not have permission under this license to share adapted material derived from this chapter or parts of it.

The images or other third party material in this chapter are included in the chapter's Creative Commons license, unless indicated otherwise in a credit line to the material. If material is not included in the chapter's Creative Commons license and your intended use is not permitted by statutory regulation or exceeds the permitted use, you will need to obtain permission directly from the copyright holder.

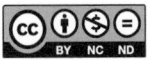

Facial Nerve Palsy (CN7)

Reuben Foo, Shweta Singhal, and Umapathi Thirugnanam

History

- Time of onset
- Symptoms: facial asymmetry, difficulty chewing/speaking/drooling, eye redness/tearing/discomfort/blurring of vision, dry eyes, inability to close eyes
- Ensure this is an isolated CN VII palsy without other systemic sensorimotor symptoms that might suggest a stroke!
- History of parotid/ear surgery
- History of trauma (temporal bone fractures/facial wounds)
- History of herpes zoster infection involving CN IX +/− VIII, i.e. external auditory canal and soft palate (Ramsay Hunt syndrome), history of recent ear infections, e.g. acute otitis media
- History of malignancy/symptoms of head and neck malignancy
- Bilateral facial nerve palsies: Consider Lyme disease, Guillain-Barre syndrome, diabetes, sarcoidosis, Parkinson's disease, multiple sclerosis, bulbar palsy.

Examination

- Ensure no long tract signs are present to suggest a stroke or intracranial tumour
- Check CN VII function to ascertain whether upper (sparing forehead) or lower (involving forehead) motor neuron lesion
- Look for possible cause:
  - Cerebellopontine angle lesion: check corneo facial sensation (CN V palsy), extraocular motility (CN VI palsy), hearing (CN VIII impairment), Brun's nystagmus
  - Temporal bone fracture: Battle sign, CSF otorrhoea
  - Ear: vesicles (Ramsay Hunt syndrome), infection
  - Parotid gland: scars, masses that suggest malignancy
  - Bell's palsy: idiopathic
- Look for possible complications:
  - Orbicularis strength, incomplete blinking
  - Lagophthalmos, exposure keratopathy (check corneal sensation and corneal staining), Bell's reflex
  - Lower lid ectropion, tearing
  - Brow ptosis
  - Chronic: ocular-oral synkinesis (inverse Marcus-Gunn jaw winking), gustatory lacrimation (crocodile tear syndrome), hemifacial spasm
- Complete ocular examination, including assessing CN II-VIII, slit lamp, and dilated fundus examination, is mandatory

Investigations

- Urgent neuroimaging if upper motor neuron lesion or multiple cranial nerve involvement is present
- Consider further imaging if temporal bone fracture or malignancy is suspected—usually warrants assessment by other specialties as well, e.g. otolaryngology, head and neck surgery

Treatment

- Refer to other specialties as required, e.g. otolaryngology if Bell's palsy/hearing affected/ear lesions
- Consider oral steroids and acyclovir for acute onset Bell's palsy
- Treatment of complications—depends on severity and predicted duration of symptoms
- Exposure keratopathy:
  - Mild: conservative management with lubricants, lid taping
  - Severe: Moist chamber, tarsorrhaphy, upper lid Botox injections, punctal plugs, surgery, e.g. upper lid gold/platinum weight implantation
  - Refer to the oculoplastics team within 2 months if the patient fails conservative management.
- Synkinesis/hemifacial spasm: Botox injections
- Brow ptosis/lower lid ectropion/facial asymmetry: surgery

GEH Perspectives

Know the Difference: It is essential to distinguish between upper motor neuron and lower motor neuron involvement when evaluating an isolated CN VII palsy. This distinction can significantly impact your diagnosis and treatment approach.

Consider Bell's Palsy: While Bell's palsy is the most common cause of isolated unilateral CN VII palsy, it's important to keep an open mind and exclude other potential causes. Always assess the patient's history and symptoms to ensure a comprehensive evaluation.

Open Access This chapter is licensed under the terms of the Creative Commons Attribution-NonCommercial-NoDerivatives 4.0 International License (http://creativecommons.org/licenses/by-nc-nd/4.0/), which permits any non-commercial use, sharing, distribution and reproduction in any medium or format, as long as you give appropriate credit to the original author(s) and the source, provide a link to the Creative Commons license and indicate if you modified the licensed material. You do not have permission under this license to share adapted material derived from this chapter or parts of it.

The images or other third party material in this chapter are included in the chapter's Creative Commons license, unless indicated otherwise in a credit line to the material. If material is not included in the chapter's Creative Commons license and your intended use is not permitted by statutory regulation or exceeds the permitted use, you will need to obtain permission directly from the copyright holder.

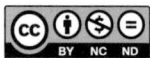

Paediatric Emergency: Leukocoria

Lim Sing Hui and Audrey Chia

History

- Parental description of a white appearance in the pupil
  - Duration, Change. Past examinations/treatments
  - History of trauma or inflammation
- Abnormal visual behaviour (e.g. roving eye movements, oculodigital reflex)
- Squint, especially esotropia
- Past medical history (e.g. malignancy, prematurity, maternal illnesses during pregnancy)
- Family history of retinoblastoma or cataracts

Examination

- Visual acuity (BE), pupil response, and relative afferent pupil defect
- Orthoptic assessment: Strabismus (cover-test) and eye movements
- Ocular examination to identify site of lesion—lens, vitreous, retina

---

L. S. Hui · A. Chia (✉)
Singapore National Eye Centre, Singapore Eye Research Institute, Singapore, Singapore
e-mail: audrey.chia.w.l@singhealth.com.sg

© The Author(s) 2026
A. C S Tan et al. (eds.), *The Global Eye Health Handbook*,
https://doi.org/10.1007/978-981-96-8861-6_41

- Cornea (haze/opacity) and anterior chamber (depth cells, hypopyon)
- Intraocular pressure (? raised)
- Lens clarity/opacity (unilateral/bilateral, morphology)
- Vitreous—clear or occupied
- Retina—mass, detachment, abnormalities (e.g. coloboma)

Investigations

- Imaging
  - Photos—external eye or fundus
  - Ultrasound B-scan to exclude retinal masses or posterior segment abnormalities when there is no/poor fundal view
  - MRI brain and orbits if suspicious for retinoblastoma (external spread)

Treatment

- Inform consultant on call for review.
  - Immediately for cases of retinoblastoma or other intraocular malignancies
  - Within days for cases of paediatric cataracts
- Other causes of leukocoria should be managed according to suspected diagnosis.

> **GEH Perspectives**
> - *Leukocoria needs urgent attention*: The appearance of leukocoria can signal serious, life- or sight-threatening conditions, so it's important to arrange an urgent review with an ophthalmologist. Early detection can make all the difference!

- *Key conditions to rule out*:
  - *Cataracts*: Early surgery can be very beneficial in some cases, so catching it early gives the best chance for improved vision.
  - *Retinoblastoma*: This can spread rapidly, and if it extends outside the eye, the risk to life increases. Early diagnosis and treatment are critical.
- *Other possible causes*: Leukocoria can also be caused by retinal issues like *retinal detachment*, *coats' disease*, or large *colobomas*. These conditions also need thorough evaluation to ensure timely management.

Open Access This chapter is licensed under the terms of the Creative Commons Attribution-NonCommercial-NoDerivatives 4.0 International License (http://creativecommons.org/licenses/by-nc-nd/4.0/), which permits any non-commercial use, sharing, distribution and reproduction in any medium or format, as long as you give appropriate credit to the original author(s) and the source, provide a link to the Creative Commons license and indicate if you modified the licensed material. You do not have permission under this license to share adapted material derived from this chapter or parts of it.

The images or other third party material in this chapter are included in the chapter's Creative Commons license, unless indicated otherwise in a credit line to the material. If material is not included in the chapter's Creative Commons license and your intended use is not permitted by statutory regulation or exceeds the permitted use, you will need to obtain permission directly from the copyright holder.

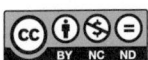

Paediatric Emergency: Non-accidental Injury (NAI): Shaken Baby Syndrome

Lim Sing Hui and Audrey Chia

History

- History not matching severity of eye findings from caregivers
- History of previous hospitalizations or injury
- Poor feeding, seizures, failure to thrive, vomiting, loss of consciousness

Examination

Watch for:

- Unstable vital signs, including bradycardia, hypothermia, hypo- or hypertension, respiratory distress, and coma
- Bruises of varying age
- Reduced visual function and RAPD
- Bilateral diffuse pre-, intra-, and subretinal haemorrhages, VH and cotton wool spots
- Occasionally blood-filled retinal schisis cavity and ring-shaped retinal folds
- Disc oedema

Investigations

- Retinal photographs
- MRI in cases of suspected raised intracranial pressure or decrease level of consciousness
- Systemic workup in collaboration with paediatrics service
- Notification of child protection agency

Treatment

- Inform consultant-on-call immediately for any case of suspected abusive head trauma with ocular signs
- Co-manage systemic injuries with paediatrics team

> **GEH Perspectives**
> - *NAI is Serious*: Non-accidental injury (NAI) carries a high risk of morbidity and mortality, so it's crucial to act quickly if you suspect it. Do not hesitate to involve the relevant nursing and medical team heads immediately. In some cases, the child may need to be admitted for observation, and it is important not to leave them alone with their caregivers.
> - *Handle Conversations Carefully*: When discussing your findings with caregivers, avoid speculating about the possible causes of the eye issues. It is best to explain that you are part of a medical team, and your findings are just one piece of a bigger clinical picture. This helps avoid misunderstandings and keeps the focus on the child's well-being.
> - *Thorough Documentation*: Make sure to document all your eye findings in detail, and if possible, capture images of the eye or retina. This helps with accurate diagnosis and follow-up, and it is important for any legal considerations.

- *Suspicious Signs*: Retinal haemorrhages at different levels in a child under 1 year old are particularly suspicious. However, keep in mind that there are other potential causes of diffuse retinal haemorrhages in infants and young children, like Terson syndrome, Purtscher retinopathy, central retinal vein occlusion (CRVO), or underlying conditions like leukaemia or bleeding disorders.

Open Access This chapter is licensed under the terms of the Creative Commons Attribution-NonCommercial-NoDerivatives 4.0 International License (http://creativecommons.org/licenses/by-nc-nd/4.0/), which permits any non-commercial use, sharing, distribution and reproduction in any medium or format, as long as you give appropriate credit to the original author(s) and the source, provide a link to the Creative Commons license and indicate if you modified the licensed material. You do not have permission under this license to share adapted material derived from this chapter or parts of it.

The images or other third party material in this chapter are included in the chapter's Creative Commons license, unless indicated otherwise in a credit line to the material. If material is not included in the chapter's Creative Commons license and your intended use is not permitted by statutory regulation or exceeds the permitted use, you will need to obtain permission directly from the copyright holder.

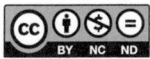

Paediatric Emergency: Allergic Conjunctivitis

Lim Sing Hui and Audrey Chia

History

- History of atopy (e.g. allergic rhinitis, eczema, drug/food allergies, etc.)
- Itching, mucoid discharge, red eye
- Allergen exposure (e.g. pets, soft toys, nearby construction site)

Examination

- Check VA which may be reduced if corneal involved
- Look for: Periocular oedema and erythema, eczematous changes
- Conjunctival hyperaemia, chemosis, tarsal follicles/papillae/giant papillae
- Limbitis/Horner-Trantas dots
- Corneal PEEs and shield ulcers (often superior location)
- Check IOP (esp if on steroids)
- Exclude retinal breaks, detachment, and dialysis (rare)

L. S. Hui · A. Chia (✉)
Singapore National Eye Centre, Singapore Eye Research Institute, Singapore, Singapore
e-mail: audrey.chia.w.l@singhealth.com.sg

© The Author(s) 2026
A. C S Tan et al. (eds.), *The Global Eye Health Handbook*,
https://doi.org/10.1007/978-981-96-8861-6_43

Investigations

- Photographs in severe cases if available/child able to cooperate

Treatment

- Allergen avoidance and advice.
- Cool compresses and avoidance of rubbing.
- Topical antihistamines, mast cell stabilisers, preservative-free lubricants.
- Cover with topical antibiotics (if corneal ulceration present).
- Topical steroids, steroid-sparing agents (e.g. Tricolimus, cyclosporin), and oral antihistamine in more severe cases.
- Referral to Paediatrics for management of systemic atopy in selected cases (or otolaryngology team for allergic rhinitis).

> **GEH Perspectives**
> - *Allergic Conjunctivitis Varies*: It can range from mild to very severe, so it's important to assess each case individually and provide the appropriate treatment and advice based on the severity of symptoms.
> - *Look for Other Allergies*: Children with allergic conjunctivitis often have other allergic symptoms, like issues with their nose, skin, or airways. Keep an eye out for these as they can help guide overall management.
> - *Check the Upper Lids*: Always remember to evert the upper lids to look for tarsal papillae, and use staining to assess the health of the cornea and check for any signs of ulceration. This is especially important in more severe cases.
> - *Recurrence is Common*: Allergic conjunctivitis tends to come back, but the good news is that symptoms often improve as children reach their teenage years.

GEH Clinical Perspectives for Paediatric Ophthalmology

- Paediatric examination takes several keys: be observant, quick, and flexible. Children have short attention spans and it is important to complete the examination efficiently.
- Use a good fixation target such as a large and bright toy. Children are usually uncooperative and have a difficult time fixating.
- Perform the less invasive examination first to avoid the child crying/struggling. Use light last as it can be distressing to some children.
- Involve the parents. Ensure that they are in the room and able to comfort the child.
- Essential components of a paediatric eye examination:
  - Vision assessment
  - Ocular alignment and motility
  - Pupils
  - Red reflex
  - External ocular examination
  - Anterior and posterior segment examination

Open Access This chapter is licensed under the terms of the Creative Commons Attribution-NonCommercial-NoDerivatives 4.0 International License (http://creativecommons.org/licenses/by-nc-nd/4.0/), which permits any non-commercial use, sharing, distribution and reproduction in any medium or format, as long as you give appropriate credit to the original author(s) and the source, provide a link to the Creative Commons license and indicate if you modified the licensed material. You do not have permission under this license to share adapted material derived from this chapter or parts of it.

The images or other third party material in this chapter are included in the chapter's Creative Commons license, unless indicated otherwise in a credit line to the material. If material is not included in the chapter's Creative Commons license and your intended use is not permitted by statutory regulation or exceeds the permitted use, you will need to obtain permission directly from the copyright holder.

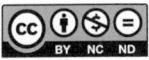

Part III

A Clinical Guide to Ocular Emergencies and Common Ocular Conditions: Other Important Conditions and Skills

Examination of Paediatric Patients

44

Lim Sing Hui and Audrey Chia

History

- Detailed history from adult/caregiver
- Suspect trauma in cases of red or painful eyes
- Medical history (including birth and development, comorbidities, family history)
- Determine vaccination and fasting status

Examination

- Document VA in each eye using an age-appropriate method
  - Preverbal: fixation and following, and reaching out for objects; preferential looking charts
  - Verbal: matching picture/letter charts; Snellen charts
- Assess corneal light reflexes (presence of strabismus)
- Check for pupil size and responses
- Orthoptic assessment: check for strabismus, limitation eye movement, or nystagmus
- External eye and dilated eye examinations

L. S. Hui · A. Chia (✉)
Singapore National Eye Centre, Singapore Eye Research Institute, Singapore, Singapore
e-mail: audrey.chia.w.l@singhealth.com.sg

Investigations

- Refraction; consider cycloplegic using:
  - <6 months: Cyclomydril every 5 minutes × 2–3
  - Cyclopentolate 0.5%–1% every 5 min × 2–3; Phenylephrine 2.5% ×1
- Ocular or Brain/Orbital images as required.

Treatment

- Refer paediatric ophthalmologist, paediatrician if needed
- Consult with pharmacist regarding age and weight adjusted dosing of medications if required

> **GEH Perspectives**
> - *Start with a Good History*: A detailed history can really help guide the rest of the examination and any necessary investigations. It's often the key to understanding what's going on with your paediatric patient.
> - *Make It Fun*: Whenever possible, try to turn the examination into a playful experience. Engaging children through play can make them more comfortable and cooperative, helping you get the information you need without causing distress.
> - *Save the Tough Stuff for Last*: Leave any potentially uncomfortable or painful parts of the exam—Like touching the lids, using eye drops, or bright lights—Until the very end. Once a child starts crying, it's hard to get their cooperation back, so try to save those steps for when absolutely necessary.
> - *Consider Sedation When Needed*: In cases where a child is uncooperative, like for foreign body removal or a thorough examination, consider using sedation with the help of an emergency physician. It can make the process smoother and less stressful for everyone.

- *General Anaesthesia for Serious Cases*: If you suspect a penetrating globe injury, it's a good idea to consider examining the child under general anaesthesia. It ensures a thorough and safe evaluation without causing unnecessary discomfort.

Open Access This chapter is licensed under the terms of the Creative Commons Attribution-NonCommercial-NoDerivatives 4.0 International License (http://creativecommons.org/licenses/by-nc-nd/4.0/), which permits any non-commercial use, sharing, distribution and reproduction in any medium or format, as long as you give appropriate credit to the original author(s) and the source, provide a link to the Creative Commons license and indicate if you modified the licensed material. You do not have permission under this license to share adapted material derived from this chapter or parts of it.

The images or other third party material in this chapter are included in the chapter's Creative Commons license, unless indicated otherwise in a credit line to the material. If material is not included in the chapter's Creative Commons license and your intended use is not permitted by statutory regulation or exceeds the permitted use, you will need to obtain permission directly from the copyright holder.

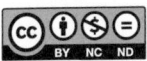

A Global Health Approach to Refractive Errors in Children and Adults

Bryan Sim and Audrey Chia

Introduction

- Refractive errors, including myopia, hyperopia, and astigmatism, are significant contributors to reversible blindness in the developing world.
- Despite being easily correctable with glasses, contact lenses, or refractive surgery, millions of people in these regions remain visually impaired due to limited access to eye care services and corrective lenses.
- Global resource limitation and lack of awareness means that many individuals, especially in rural and underserved communities, suffer from impaired vision that affects their quality of life, education, and economic opportunities [1–3].
- Addressing refractive errors through affordable and accessible eye care is crucial in reducing the burden of preventable blindness and improving overall well-being in the developing world.
- Globally, refractive errors and cataracts are the primary contributors to vision impairment and blindness.
- Uncorrected refractive error continues to be a major cause of vision impairment across all countries, affecting both children and adults.

B. Sim · A. Chia (✉)
Singapore National Eye Centre, Singapore Eye Research Institute, Singapore, Singapore
e-mail: audrey.chia.w.l@singhealth.com.sg

© The Author(s) 2026
A. C S Tan et al. (eds.), *The Global Eye Health Handbook*,
https://doi.org/10.1007/978-981-96-8861-6_45

Types of Common Refractive Errors Encountered in Developing and Developed Countries

	EMMETROPIA	MYOPIA	HYPEROPIA	ASTIGMATISM	PRESBYOPIA
DESCRIPTION	Normal refractive condition of the eye. Light rays are focused on the retina when the accommodation is relaxed.	Axial length is longer than eye's total refractive power. Light rays are focused in front of the retina when the accommodation is relaxed.	Axial length is shorter than eye's total refractive power. Light rays are focused behind the retina when the accommodation is relaxed.	The curvature of the cornea and/or crystalline lens is not spherical, resulting in light rays focusing on two different focal points.	Occurs when the lens gradually loses the ability to focus clearly on different distances, especially at near.
SYMPTOMS	Clear vision at all distances	Distance vision blur	Near vision blur. If severe (more than +4.00D), distance vision may be affected as well.	Both distance and near vision may be affected	Near vision blur
OPTICAL CORRECTION	No correction required	Concave lens	Convex lens	Cylindrical lens	Reading glasses for near work

Credits: Myopia Online Course, SNEC Myopia Service

Classification of Myopia: Qualitative definitions	
Axial myopia	A myopic refractive state resulting from a greater than normal axial length.
Refractive myopia	A myopic refractive state due to changes in the structure or location of the image forming structures of the eye, i.e. the *cornea and lens*
Secondary myopia	A myopic refractive state due to drug, glaucoma, corneal disease, e.g. keratoconus or systemic clinical syndrome that can be identified

Quantitative definitions (International Myopia Institute (IMI))	
Pre-myopia	*Spherical equivalent (SE)* $\leq$ +0.75D and > −0.50D in children with risk factors for myopia development
Myopia	*Spherical equivalent (SE)* $\leq$ −0.50D
Low myopia	*Spherical equivalent (SE)* $\leq$ −0.50D and > −6.00D
High myopia	*Spherical equivalent (SE)* $\leq$ −6.00D

History

- Symptoms: blurred distance vision (myopia), blurred near vision (hyperopia, presbyopia), seeing glare or halos around lights (astigmatism)
- Onset: Gradual
- In children:
  - Unable to see whiteboard in school
  - Squinting while doing homework, reading or watching TV
  - Abnormal head posture
  - Frequent rubbing, blinking of eyes, eye fatigue
  - Holding reading material closer/sitting closer to view objects
- Any glasses wear, age of first spectacle correction
- Risk factors for myopia:
  - Non-modifiable: family history of myopia
  - Modifiable: amount of outdoor time, near work

- Any pre-existing myopia control intervention, e.g. atropine eyedrops, myopia control glasses or contact lenses
- Any other risk factors for syndromic causes of myopia, e.g.
  - Stickler syndrome classically inherited in an autosomal dominant fashion—strong family history of retinal detachment or
  - Primary congenital glaucoma (PCG): mostly sporadic, 10–40% are familial, with an autosomal recessive inheritance—family history of glaucoma

Examination

- Gold standard is manifest or cycloplegic refraction.
- Vision will improve with pinhole.
- Clinical exam.
  - Signs of a myopic fundus (more common in older children/adults):
    - Tilted disc
    - Peripapillary atrophy (PPA)
    - Posterior staphyloma
    - Myopic macular degeneration (MMD): tessellated fundus, chorioretinal atrophy (diffuse/patchy)
    - Plus signs: Foster-Fuchs spots, lacquer cracks, haemorrhages suggestive of myopia choroidal neovascularisation (mCNV)
    - *Assess for ocular associations*:
      - Retinopathy of prematurity (ROP)
      - Albinism
      - Congenital glaucoma
      - Congenital stationary night blindness (CSNB)
      - Ectopia lentis
      - Retinitis pigmentosa (RP) (bony spicules)
      - *To rule out complications of myopia*:
        - Cataract (nuclear sclerosis)
        - Intraocular pressure (IOP) (glaucoma), cup disc ratio (CDR)

- Dilated fundal exam: Macular hole, epiretinal membrane (ERM), retinal tear/detachment
- Myopic strabismus fixus
- *To look for any systemic associations*:
  - Down's syndrome (Trisomy 21)
    - Upslanting palpebral fissures
    - Epicanthal folds
    - Clinodactyly
    - Intellectual disability, developmental delays
    - Obesity
  - Ehlers-Danlos syndrome (EDS)
    - Joint hypermobility (frequent joint dislocations, sprains, and subluxations)
    - Skin hyperextensibility
    - Strabismus, amblyopia, irregular astigmatism
  - Marfan syndrome (MFS)
    - Tall Stature, arachnodactyly
    - Chest *d*eformities: Pectus excavatum (a sunken chest) or pectus carinatum (a protruding chest)
    - Scoliosis: Abnormal curvature of the spine (scoliosis) is common and can be severe in some cases.
    - Joint *h*ypermobility
    - Mitral valve prolapse (MVP)
  - Stickler syndrome (STL)
    - Sensorineural hearing loss
    - Pierre Robin Sequence
    - Ocular: Retinal detachment (RD), Cataracts, and Glaucoma
  - Alport syndrome
    - Progressive kidney disease
    - Sensorineural hearing loss
    - Ocular: Anterior Lenticonus, dot-and-fleck retinopathy

Refractive error	Possible causes or associations
Myopia	Congenital stationary night blindness (CSNB)
	Cataract (index myopia)
	Keratoconus
	Retinitis pigmentosa (RP)
	Glaucoma (primary congenital glaucoma (PCG))
	Albinism
	Blue cone dystrophy
	Lens subluxation
	Retinopathy of prematurity (ROP)
	Myopia of prematurity (MOP)
	Weill-Marchesani syndrome
	Microspherophakia
	Marfan syndrome (MFS)
	Ehlers-Danlos syndrome (EDS)
	Down syndrome
	Stickler syndrome
	Alport syndrome
	Diabetes Mellitus (uncontrolled)
Astigmatism	RP
	Albinism
	Lens subluxation
	Keratoconus
	Marfan syndrome (MFS)
	Ehlers-Danlos syndrome (EDS)
	Down syndrome
	Alport syndrome
High hyperopia	Leber congenital amaurosis (LCA)
	Albinism
	Achromatopsia
	Down syndrome

Investigations

- Refraction as above
- Optical coherence tomography (OCT): to confirm diagnosis for above complications—macula hole, epiretinal membrane (ERM), posterior staphyloma, choroidal neovascularisation (CNV), dome-shaped macula

- Fundus fluorescein angiography (FFA) and OCT-angiography to further delineate choroidal neovascular membrane (CNV) (classic pattern of leakage)

Interventions for childhood myopia control		
1	Environmental Modifications: *Increased Outdoor Time/Less near work*	
	Mechanism	Increased exposure to sunlight and the outdoor environment has been associated with a lower incidence of myopia onset and slower progression in children. Natural light exposure helps regulate dopamine release in the retina, which may inhibit excessive axial length growth, a key factor in myopia development.
	Implementation	Public health initiatives can promote outdoor activities in schools and communities. Recommendations often include encouraging at least 2 h of outdoor play per day for children.
	Advantages	Cost-effective and freely available. Provides additional health benefits, such as physical fitness and mental well-being.
	Challenges	Difficult to monitor and reinforce consistent outdoor time. Urban environments may have limited safe spaces for outdoor activities.
2	Pharmacological therapy (Atropine) [4]	
	Mechanism	Low-dose atropine eye drops (typically 0.01–0.05%) are used to slow the progression of myopia. The mechanism of atropine is unknown—Theories include: Retina, choroid, sclera remodelling
	Implementation	Typically administered as one drop in each eye before bedtime. Treatment duration and dosage may vary based on the child's response and myopia progression.
	Advantages	Proven efficacy in significantly slowing myopia progression in numerous clinical studies. (ATOM1/2, LAMP studies) Can be combined with other myopia control strategies for enhanced effect

Interventions for childhood myopia control

	Challenges	Potential side effects include glare and near blur, though these are minimized with low-dose atropine. Requires regular monitoring and follow-up Access and affordability may be limited in some regions
3	Myopia control glasses (DIMS and HALT lenses) [4]	
	Mechanism	DIMS (Defocus Incorporated Multiple Segments) and HALT (Highly Aspherical L enslet Target) lenses are specially designed glasses that create a myopic defocus on the peripheral retina while providing clear central vision. This defocus is thought to slow the elongation of the eyeball, which is responsible for myopia progression.
	Implementation	These lenses are worn full time for refractive correction and myopia control.
	Advantages	Non-invasive and easy to use. Proven to effectively slow myopia progression in clinical trials.
	Challenges	Higher cost compared to standard single-vision lenses. Limited availability in some regions. Compliance can be an issue if children are reluctant to wear glasses, e.g. in low myopes
4	Myopia Control Multifocal Contact Lenses [4]	
	Mechanism	These contact lenses are designed with multiple zones of focus, creating a similar myopic defocus which helps slow the progression of myopia
	Implementation	These lenses are prescribed by an eye care professional and need to be worn consistently, typically on a daily wear schedule. They are ideal for older children and teenagers who are comfortable with contact lens use.
	Advantages	Effective in slowing myopia progression. Provides a glasses-free option, which can be preferable for active children.
	Challenges	Requires proper hygiene and care to prevent infective keratitis Not suitable for very young children. Higher cost and need for regular replacement. Availability may be limited in certain areas.

Interventions for childhood myopia control	
5	Orthokeratology (Ortho-K or OK) lenses [4]	
Mechanism	*Corneal reshaping:* Ortho-K lenses temporarily reshape the cornea, particularly flattening the central cornea, to correct myopia. *Peripheral defocus theory:* One key mechanism believed to contribute to myopia control is the induction of peripheral myopic defocus.
Implementation	*Overnight lens Wear:* The child wears the Ortho-K lenses overnight to reshape the cornea. Upon waking, the lenses are removed, and the child can see clearly throughout the day without additional corrective lenses. *Regular monitoring:* Regular follow-up visits are crucial to monitor the fit of the lenses, corneal health, and the progression of myopia. Adjustments to the lenses may be needed as the child's eyes grow and change.
Advantages	Slows childhood myopia progression Offers a non-invasive, reversible alternative to refractive surgery, making it a safer option for children. Daytime freedom from glasses (without the need for daytime glasses or contact lenses)
Challenges	Compliance and commitment: Consistent nightly wear of Ortho-K lenses is essential for effective myopia control. Irregular use can lead to inconsistent vision correction and reduced efficacy in slowing myopia progression. Risk of infective keratitis: Particularly if hygiene practices are not strictly adhered to. Parents and children must be diligent in cleaning and storing the lenses properly. High cost Limited availability: Access to qualified practitioners and specialized Ortho-K lenses may be limited in some areas, making it less accessible for some children. Risk of rebound myopia when lenses stopped

Global Eye Health (GEH) Tips for Clinicians

1. *Provision of accurate and appropriate refractive correction to prevent amblyopia*
   - Screening for refractive errors like astigmatism, hyperopia, and myopia is recommended, as it is a leading cause of reversible blindness that is easily correctable
   - Reduced visual acuity from refractive error can be effectively corrected with spectacles and contact lenses and, less commonly, intraocular lens and laser refractive surgery
   - Ensure Accurate Prescription: Provide the child with the most accurate refractive correction possible. This is crucial because proper vision correction can significantly improve the child's quality of life and educational outcomes. Emphasise the importance of wearing the prescribed glasses consistently, particularly for children with astigmatism or significant myopia/hyperopia, to prevent amblyopia or other complications.
   - Educate the child and their caregivers on the importance of refractive correction as a reversible form of vision loss. Explain that, unlike many other eye conditions, the vision impairment caused by refractive errors can often be fully corrected with appropriate lenses.
2. *Preventing the onset and progression of childhood myopia*
   - Increasing outdoor time and reducing near work may delay the onset and progression of myopia
   - Various treatment modalities offer various approaches to managing childhood myopia, each with its advantages and challenges. A combination of strategies tailored to the child's needs, environment, and access to resources is often the most effective approach to slowing the progression of myopia.
3. *Rule of potentially life and sight-threatening associations of refractive errors*
   - Always perform an IOP check and formal dilated fundus examination to assess for glaucomatous optic neuropathy in a child presenting with myopia, as it may signify congenital glaucoma which can be treated with glaucoma medications and early surgical intervention

- Early identification can prevent intractable blindness which will impact a child's overall quality of life
- Besides IOP, ensure that the child is screened for other conditions like strabismus, amblyopia, or keratoconus, which can often accompany or complicate myopia and astigmatism.
- Treat underlying cause of refractive error e.g. allergic eye disease causing keratoconus resulting in high astigmatism/myopia with antihistamine eye drops and avoidance of eye rubbing

References

1. GBD 2019 Blindness and Vision Impairment Collaborators; Vision Loss Expert Group of the Global Burden of Disease Study. Causes of blindness and vision impairment in 2020 and trends over 30 years, and prevalence of avoidable blindness in relation to VISION 2020: the Right to Sight: an analysis for the Global Burden of Disease Study. Lancet Glob Health. 2021 Feb;9(2):e144–e160. https://doi.org/10.1016/S2214-109X(20)30489-7.
2. Fricke, TR, Tahhan N, Resnikoff S, Papas E, Burnett A, Suit MH, Naduvilath T, Naidoo K, Global Prevalence of Presbyopia and Vision Impairment from Uncorrected Presbyopia: Systematic Review, Meta-analysis, and Modelling, Ophthalmology. 2018 May 9.
3. Burton MJ, Ramke J, Marques AP, Bourne RR, Congdon N, Jones I, et al. The Lancet Global Health commission on Global Eye Health: vision beyond 2020. Lancet Glob Health. 2021; 9(4):e489–e551.
4. Bullimore MA, Saunders KJ, Baraas RC, Berntsen DA, Chen Z, Chia AWL, Goto S, Jiang J, Lan W, Logan NS, Najjar RP, Polling JR, Read SA, Woodman-Pieterse EC, Széll N, Verkicharla PK, Wu PC, Zhu X, Loughman J, Nagra M, Phillips JR, Tran HDM, Vera-Diaz FA, Yam J, Liu YM, Singh SE, Wildsoet CF. IMI—Interventions for Controlling Myopia Onset and Progression 2025. Invest. Ophthalmol. Vis. Sci. 2025;66(12):39.

Open Access This chapter is licensed under the terms of the Creative Commons Attribution-NonCommercial-NoDerivatives 4.0 International License (http://creativecommons.org/licenses/by-nc-nd/4.0/), which permits any noncommercial use, sharing, distribution and reproduction in any medium or format, as long as you give appropriate credit to the original author(s) and the source, provide a link to the Creative Commons license and indicate if you modified the licensed material. You do not have permission under this license to share adapted material derived from this chapter or parts of it.

The images or other third party material in this chapter are included in the chapter's Creative Commons license, unless indicated otherwise in a credit line to the material. If material is not included in the chapter's Creative Commons license and your intended use is not permitted by statutory regulation or exceeds the permitted use, you will need to obtain permission directly from the copyright holder.

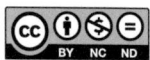

Cataract 46

Yap Guan Hui and Melissa Wong

History

- Blurred vision at distance or near
- Glare (difficulty seeing in bright lights or haloes or streaks around lights)
- Difficulty seeing in low light situations (including poor night vision)
- Loss of contrast sensitivity
- Loss of ability to discern colours
- Worsening near-sightedness or change in refractive status ("second sight" phenomenon)
- *Risk factors*:
- Modifiable: Diabetes mellitus, steroid use, ultraviolet exposure, smoking
- Non-modifiable: Genetic predisposition (family history), previous trauma or surgery or radiation, ocular diseases (e.g. retinitis pigmentosa, uveitis)

Examination

- Slit lamp examination and dilated eye exam
- Factors affecting surgical planning: type and density of the cataract, size of the dilated pupil, cornea clarity, presence of corneal guttata/Fuch's endothelial dystrophy, lens stability (phacodonesis), AC depth and optic nerve and retina (affects visual prognosis)

Investigations

- Refraction
- Measurement of axial length, corneal refractive power, and AC depth
- Corneal topography and endothelial cell counts
- Ultrasound biomicroscopy if suspecting zonular laxity/zonulysis or to search for pre-existing posterior capsular breach in posterior polar cataracts

Management Tips

- Planning strategy and technique of cataract surgery for each case (especially challenging ones) and anticipating equipment needed and potential complications is key in optimising good outcomes.
- Every step of the surgery matters! The success of each step gives rise to much higher chances of success of the subsequent steps. For starters in cataract surgery, always ensure that every step of the surgery is done correctly to minimise jeopardising the subsequent steps.
- Always maintain honest and open communications with the patient—advise the patient of relevant risks of the surgery, and potential other relevant risks pertaining to the patient's cataract and visual prognosis. Good counselling will minimise unrealistic expectations and unhappy patients.

GEH Perspectives

- *Prevention Matters*: Slowing the development of cataracts can be as simple as recommending some preventive steps. Encourage wearing good-quality UV-blocking sunglasses to reduce UV exposure and using protective eyewear to prevent injuries. If your patient has diabetes, suggest maintaining good control of blood sugar levels. Also, letting patients know that quitting smoking can help reduce the progression of cataracts is a great tip for long-term eye health!

- *Surgery is the Solution*: When cataracts start to affect vision, surgery is the way to go. Depending on local resources, refer patients for the most suitable option—whether it's phacoemulsification, extracapsular cataract extraction, or manual small incision cataract surgery. Each approach works well in different settings, so finding the right expertise ensures the best care for your patients.

Open Access This chapter is licensed under the terms of the Creative Commons Attribution-NonCommercial-NoDerivatives 4.0 International License (http://creativecommons.org/licenses/by-nc-nd/4.0/), which permits any non-commercial use, sharing, distribution and reproduction in any medium or format, as long as you give appropriate credit to the original author(s) and the source, provide a link to the Creative Commons license and indicate if you modified the licensed material. You do not have permission under this license to share adapted material derived from this chapter or parts of it.

The images or other third party material in this chapter are included in the chapter's Creative Commons license, unless indicated otherwise in a credit line to the material. If material is not included in the chapter's Creative Commons license and your intended use is not permitted by statutory regulation or exceeds the permitted use, you will need to obtain permission directly from the copyright holder.

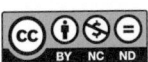

Age-Related Macular Degeneration

Charles Ong and Anna C S Tan

Classification

Early—medium drusen (between 63 and 125 microns) without pigmentary abnormalities

Intermediate—large drusen (larger than 125 microns) or medium drusen with pigmentary abnormalities

*125 microns is the average diameter of the retinal vein at the optic disc margin

Advanced—neovascular AMD (nAMD) or geographic atrophy (GA; advanced dry AMD)

C. Ong
Singapore National Eye Centre, Singapore Eye Research Institute, Singapore, Singapore

A. C S Tan (✉)
Department of Medical Retina, Singapore National Eye Centre, Singapore Eye Research Institute, Singapore, Singapore
e-mail: anna.tan.c.s@singhealth.com.sg

Early/Intermediate AMD and Geographic Atrophy (GA)

History
- Blurring of vision, poor vision in low light conditions, may be asymptomatic in early stages.

Examination
- Visual acuity
- Significant cataract (cataract surgery may be considered to optimise vision)
- Presence of drusen

Investigations
- Optical coherence tomography
- Colour photo and autofluorescence to document GA

Management
- Amsler chart monitoring.
- Patient education that there is a risk of conversion to neovascular AMD.
- Consider AREDs supplements in cases of intermediate/advanced AMD.
- Cessation of smoking.
- Intravitreal injections for GA are currently approved in the USA, to reduce disease progression; however, their use in Asian patients is still controversial.

GEH Perspectives

Follow-up needs: For patients with early or intermediate AMD, frequent visits to a tertiary service may not be necessary. Focus on patient education and encourage self-monitoring.

OCT monitoring: Keep in mind that OCT monitoring is essential for detecting early signs of disease progression in high-risk patients or conversion to neovascular AMD, even if patients aren't experiencing symptoms. Regular scans can help catch changes early.

> *When to schedule regular follow-ups*: Consider more frequent follow-ups in specific cases, such as:
>
> - Patients with advanced AMD in one eye who rely on their only seeing eye.
> - Those with rapidly progressing disease, as indicated by OCT changes.
> - Patients showing atypical features, like serous pigment epithelial detachments (PEDs).
>
> *Visual rehabilitation*: If a patient experiences significant visual impairment due to geographic atrophy (GA), do not hesitate to refer them to a visual rehabilitation service. These resources can help enhance their quality of life.

Neovascular Age-Related Macular Degeneration

- nAMD is an advanced form of AMD that can cause rapid and severe visual loss.
- Choroidal neovascularization (CNV) and polypoidal choroidal vasculopathy (PCV) are subtypes of nAMD.
- PCV has a higher incidence in Asian compared to Caucasian populations.
- CNV is further subcategorized based on anatomical layers into type 1 (sub-RPE; occult), type 2 (subretinal; classic), and type 3 (intraretinal; retinal angiomatous proliferation).

History
- Drop in vision, metamorphopsia, scotoma
- Modifiable risk factor—smoking

Examination
- VA, intraocular pressure, lens status
- Dilated fundus examination looking for signs such as:
  - Subretinal/sub-RPE haemorrhage
  - Subretinal fluid
  - Pigment epithelial detachment (PED)

- Exudates
- Subretinal fibrosis
- Orange nodule (polypoidal lesion in PCV)

Investigations

Colour Fundus Photo

OCT Macula
- Sub/intraretinal fluid
- Subretinal hyper-reflective material
  - Signifies blood, fibrin, or fibrosis
- PED
- Double layer sign may correspond to neovascular network
- Sharp peaked PED, en face OCT complex RPE elevation and sub-RPE ring like lesion (diagnostic features of PCV on OCT)

OCTA
- Visualization of flow signals and neovascular network

FFA/ICGA
- Classic CNV on FFA—early lacy hyperfluorescence with subsequent leakage
- Occult CNV on FFA—fibrovascular PED or late leakage of undetermined sources
- PCV on ICGA—polyp, branching vascular network

Management
- Stop smoking
- AREDS2 supplementation
- Home Amsler monitoring
- Intravitreal anti-VEGF injections for nAMD
- Consider combination therapy with photodynamic therapy for PCV

47 Age-Related Macular Degeneration

> **GEH Perspectives: Neovascular Age-Related Macular Degeneration (NAMD)**
>
> *Early detection and timely treatment*: Remember that NAMD is a chronic disease. Early detection, regular follow-ups, and timely intravitreal injections are crucial to prevent permanent vision loss. Encourage patients to be proactive about their eye health!
>
> *Patient education and involvement*: Take the time to counsel patients about their condition thoroughly. Make sure they understand the nature of NAMD and its potential impact on vision. Involving them in treatment decisions fosters a sense of ownership and commitment to their care.
>
> *Address barriers to treatment*: Identify any barriers that may hinder long-term treatment and adherence to intravitreal therapy (IVT). Whether it's financial, logistical, or emotional challenges, addressing these issues can significantly improve treatment outcomes and patient satisfaction (Table 47.1).

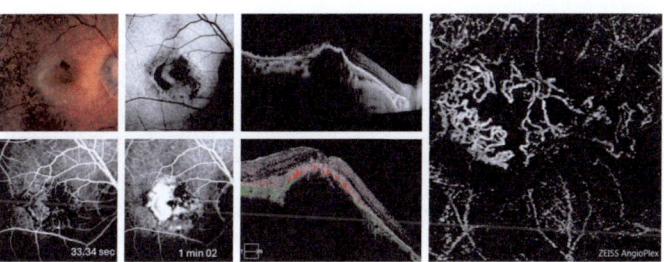

Figure above shows multi-modal imaging of neovascular AMD showing a type 2 neovascularisation (NV). Colour fundus photo (top left) shows the presence of a central macula lesion with subretinal blood, fundus autofluorescence (top row second column) shows the hyper and hypoautofluorescence in the area of NV. FFA (bottom row first and second column) below shows early lacy hyperfluorescence with late leakage. OCT (top row third column) shows area of SHRM, cross sectional OCTA (bottom row third column) show flow within the SHRM and en face OCTA shows a network of vascularisation

Table 47.1 Recommended timing and type of follow-up for various AMD stages

AMD severity	Suggested follow-up interval	Suggested disposition/right site
Early dry AMD	NA	Primary care optometrists
Intermediate dry AMD	12–18 months	Primary care optometrists Virtual eye clinics Ophthalmology clinic
Advanced dry AMD (GA)	4–6 months	Ophthalmology clinic with OCT imaging and IVT GA treatment capabilities Patients may be subsequently discharged back to primary care optometrists
Neovascular AMD	Within 2 weeks	Ophthalmology clinic with OCT imaging and IVT aVEGF capabilities

Note: Virtual eye clinics refers to consultation visits for stable patients, where imaging with wide-field fundus photography and OCT is acquired. Only patients with significant changes in their vision and OCT are seen by an ophthalmologist on the same day. The rest of the patient's photos and OCTs are graded off-line by an ophthalmologist and follow-up appointments are sent to the patient accordingly

Abbreviations: *AMD* age related macular degeneration, *aVEGF* anti-vascular endothelial growth factor, *GA* geographic atrophy, *IVT* intravitreal, *OCT* optical coherence tomography

Open Access This chapter is licensed under the terms of the Creative Commons Attribution-NonCommercial-NoDerivatives 4.0 International License (http://creativecommons.org/licenses/by-nc-nd/4.0/), which permits any non-commercial use, sharing, distribution and reproduction in any medium or format, as long as you give appropriate credit to the original author(s) and the source, provide a link to the Creative Commons license and indicate if you modified the licensed material. You do not have permission under this license to share adapted material derived from this chapter or parts of it.

The images or other third party material in this chapter are included in the chapter's Creative Commons license, unless indicated otherwise in a credit line to the material. If material is not included in the chapter's Creative Commons license and your intended use is not permitted by statutory regulation or exceeds the permitted use, you will need to obtain permission directly from the copyright holder.

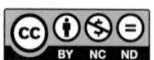

Diabetic Retinopathy

Charles Ong and Anna C S Tan

Classification

- Non-proliferative diabetic retinopathy (NPDR)
  - Mild—microaneurysms only
  - Moderate—more than microaneurysms but less than severe NPDR
  - Severe
    - 4 quadrants of haemorrhages ($\geq$ ETDRS standard photograph 2A)
    - 2 quadrants of venous beading ($\geq$ ETDRS standard photograph 6A) OR
    - 1 quadrant of intraretinal microvascular abnormalities (IRMA) ($\geq$ ETDRS standard photograph 8A)
- Proliferative diabetic retinopathy (PDR)
  - Presence of neovascularization at the disc (NVD) or elsewhere (NVE)

C. Ong
Singapore National Eye Centre, Singapore Eye Research Institute, Singapore, Singapore

A. C S Tan (✉)
Department of Medical Retina, Singapore National Eye Centre, Singapore Eye Research Institute, Singapore, Singapore
e-mail: anna.tan.c.s@singhealth.com.sg

© The Author(s) 2026
A. C S Tan et al. (eds.), *The Global Eye Health Handbook*,
https://doi.org/10.1007/978-981-96-8861-6_48

- Vision threatening complications
  - Diabetic macula oedema (DME)
  - Vitreous haemorrhage (VH)
  - Tractional retinal detachment (TRD)
  - Diabetic macula ischaemia
  - Neovascular glaucoma with neovascularization of iris (NVI)

> **Why Is a Screening Programme Important for Diabetic Retinopathy?**
> - It is an epidemiologically important health problem affecting large proportions of the population.
> - The natural history from latest to declared disease is adequately understood.
> - There is a suitable screening test—Fundus photography—That is acceptable to the population.
> - Early treatment for DR will prevent permanent vision loss from diabetic eye disease.
> - Cost of screening is balanced against the potential cost to the health system if DR is not properly screened and treated.

History

- Drop in vision, metamorphopsia, scotoma
- Diabetic treatment—medication, insulin, recent HbA1c
- Other diabetic complications such as ischaemic heart disease, foot gangrene, kidney disease
- Modifiable risk factors—smoking, diet, and exercise

Examination

- VA, intraocular pressure, lens status
- Check iris for signs of neovascularisation and consider a gonioscopy to look for neovascularisation in the angles

48 Diabetic Retinopathy

- Dilated fundus examination looking for signs such as:
  - Microaneurysms
  - Haemorrhages
  - Hard exudation
  - Macula oedema
  - Microvascular changes
  - Presence of IRMAs, NVE, NVD

Investigations

- Widefield colour fundus photo for documentation
- OCT macula to look for diabetic macula oedema
- OCTA look for peripheral areas of capillary fall out, NVEs and NVDs, and determine the foveal avascular zone
- Widefield fundus fluorescein angiography when peripheral ischaemia or neovascularisation is suspected.

Management

- Screening programme should be set up at a population level if not already established.
- Lifestyle modification—smoking cessation, weight loss, exercise.
- Co-management of diabetes and systemic risk factors with physician.
- Pan-retinal photocoagulation (PRP) for PDR.
- Consider PRP for severe NPDR in select patient groups (e.g. poor compliance, fellow eye lost to diabetic retinopathy).
- Diabetic macula oedema.
  - Foveal involvement.
    - DME with vision of 6/7.5 or better can be observed
    - DME with vision loss (6/9 or worse)
      - Intravitreal anti-VEGF injections
      - Intravitreal steroid injections
  - Extra-foveal macula oedema can be treated with focal laser.

GEH Perspectives
- Diabetes and diabetic eye disease requires screening to detect disease early to prevent permanent vision loss and long-term good diabetic control will reduce the risk of complications
- The presence of cotton wool spots, microvascular changes and inner retinal thinning seen on the OCT may be signs of an ischaemic fundus and FFA should be done to determine the extent of capillary fall out
- DME requires long term follow-up and timely IVT for the best visual outcome
- Patients should be adequately counselled about their disease and should be included in treatment decisions
- Barriers to long term treatment and adherence to IVT should be identified and addressed (Table 48.1)

Figure below shows multi-modal imaging of an eye with severe diabetic retinopathy. Widefield colour fundus photo (top left) shows the presence of haemorrhages and cotton wool spots. FFA (top row second column) shows leaking microaneurysms and patchy capillary drop-out. OCTA (top row right) shows patchy capillary drop out with a normal sized foveal avascular zone. OCT (bottom row) shows non-foveal involving macula oedema with hyper-reflective dots.

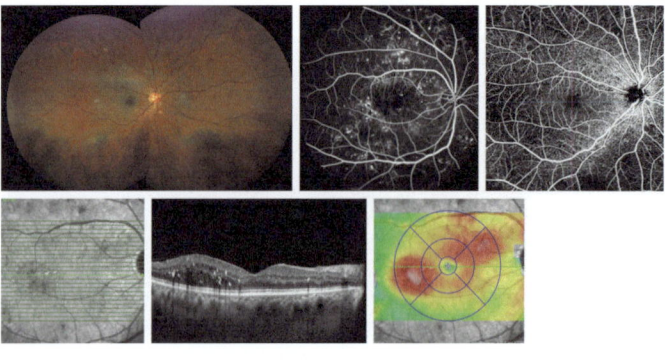

Table 48.1 Recommended timing and type of follow-up for various DR stages

DR/DME severity	Suggested follow-up interval	Suggested disposition/right site
No DR	12–18 months	Diabetic retinal photography Community eye clinic
Mild NPDR	12 months	Diabetic retinal photography Community eye clinic
Moderate NPDR	6–8 months	Ophthalmology clinic
Severe NPDR	2–4 months	Ophthalmology clinic with PRP capabilities
PDR	Within 1 month	Ophthalmology clinic with PRP and/or IVT anti VEGF capabilities
Non CIDME	4–6 months	Ophthalmology clinic with OCT imaging
CI DME with good vision (VA 6/7.5 or better)	3–4 months	Ophthalmology clinic with OCT imaging
CI DME with poor vision (VA 6/9 or worse)	Within 1 month	Ophthalmology clinic with OCT imaging with IVT anti VEGF capabilities
Diabetic vitreous haemorrhage	Within 1 month	Ophthalmology clinic with surgical retina service, PRP and/or IVT anti VEGF capabilities
Tractional retinal detachment threatening macula	At the soonest	Ophthalmology clinic with surgical retina and PRP capabilities

Note: Community eye clinics refer to primary and secondary eye care services. Diabetic retinal photography is performed in many primary health centres and is read with a combination of artificial intelligence and human graders

Abbreviations: *CI DME* Centre involving diabetic macula oedema, *DR* diabetic retinopathy, *IVT anti VEGF* intravitreal anti vascular endothelial growth factor, *NPDR* non proliferative diabetic retinopathy, *OCT* optical coherence tomography, *PRP* pan-retinal photocoagulation, *VA* visual acuity

Open Access This chapter is licensed under the terms of the Creative Commons Attribution-NonCommercial-NoDerivatives 4.0 International License (http://creativecommons.org/licenses/by-nc-nd/4.0/), which permits any noncommercial use, sharing, distribution and reproduction in any medium or format, as long as you give appropriate credit to the original author(s) and the source, provide a link to the Creative Commons license and indicate if you modified the licensed material. You do not have permission under this license to share adapted material derived from this chapter or parts of it.

The images or other third party material in this chapter are included in the chapter's Creative Commons license, unless indicated otherwise in a credit line to the material. If material is not included in the chapter's Creative Commons license and your intended use is not permitted by statutory regulation or exceeds the permitted use, you will need to obtain permission directly from the copyright holder.

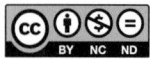

Central Serous Chorioretinopathy (CSCR) 49

Charles Ong and Anna C S Tan

History

Symptoms
- Reduction in vision
- Scotoma
- Metamorphopsia
- Dyschromatopsia
- Duration of symptoms

Risk factors
- Steroid use, supplement use, traditional medicine use
- Occupation, stress levels

C. Ong
Singapore National Eye Centre, Singapore Eye Research Institute, Singapore, Singapore
e-mail: charles.ong.j.t@snec.com.sg

A. C S Tan (✉)
Department of Medical Retina, Singapore National Eye Centre, Singapore Eye Research Institute, Singapore, Singapore
e-mail: anna.tan.c.s@singhealth.com.sg

Examination

- VA, intraocular pressure, lens status
- Dilated fundus examination looking for signs such as:
- Subretinal fluid
- PED
- Look for the presence of an optic disc pit

Investigations

- OCT macula
  - Optically empty neurosensory retina elevation (sub retinal fluid)
  - Pachychoroid (thick choroid)
  - Presence of a PED
- FFA
  - Early hyperfluorescent spot that gradually enlarges (ink blot pattern)
  - Vertical column of hyperfluorescence (smoke stack pattern)
- FAF
  - Gravitational tract in chronic CSCR

Management

- In acute CSR, observation is recommended in most cases as it is self-limiting
- Discontinue any potential offending medications, such as steroids, which can include oral, inhaled or topical administration
- Photodynamic therapy if chronic or recurrent
- Focal laser can be considered for extrafoveal origins of leakage

GEH Perspectives
- Although most CSCR will resolve spontaneously with visual acuity improvement, many patients may still experience issues with contrast sensitivity and colour vision disturbances

- Despite PDT or focal laser and the resolution of subretinal fluid, vision may not recover if there is photoreceptors dysfunction due to chronic disease
- Many traditional medicine preparations e.g. ginseng may contain steroids or steroid like components and should be avoided
- Apart from oral steroids, topical, inhaled and injected steroids can also trigger CSCR.

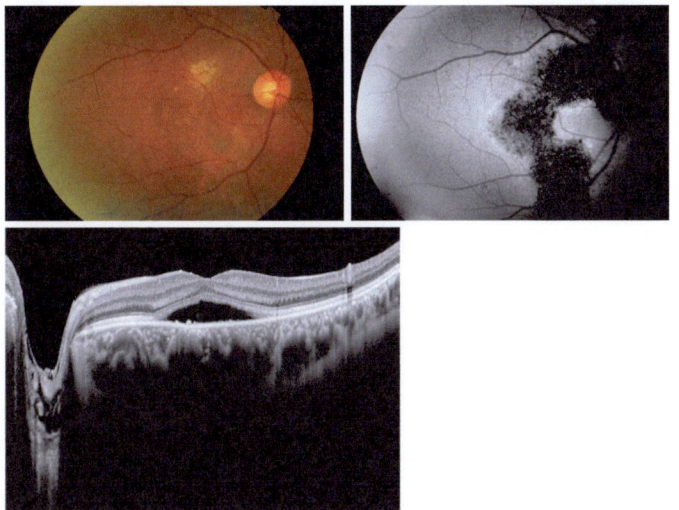

Figure above shows multimodal imaging of an eye with chronic CSCR, colour fundus photo (top left) shows macula fluid and pigmentary changes, fundus autofluorescence (top right) shows the presence of descending gravitational tracts, and OCT imaging confirms the presence of subretinal fluid.

Open Access This chapter is licensed under the terms of the Creative Commons Attribution-NonCommercial-NoDerivatives 4.0 International License (http://creativecommons.org/licenses/by-nc-nd/4.0/), which permits any noncommercial use, sharing, distribution and reproduction in any medium or format, as long as you give appropriate credit to the original author(s) and the source, provide a link to the Creative Commons license and indicate if you modified the licensed material. You do not have permission under this license to share adapted material derived from this chapter or parts of it.

The images or other third party material in this chapter are included in the chapter's Creative Commons license, unless indicated otherwise in a credit line to the material. If material is not included in the chapter's Creative Commons license and your intended use is not permitted by statutory regulation or exceeds the permitted use, you will need to obtain permission directly from the copyright holder.

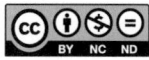

Glaucoma: Referral Pathway

Claire Peterson, Zhu Li Yap, Sahil Thakur, and Rahat Husain

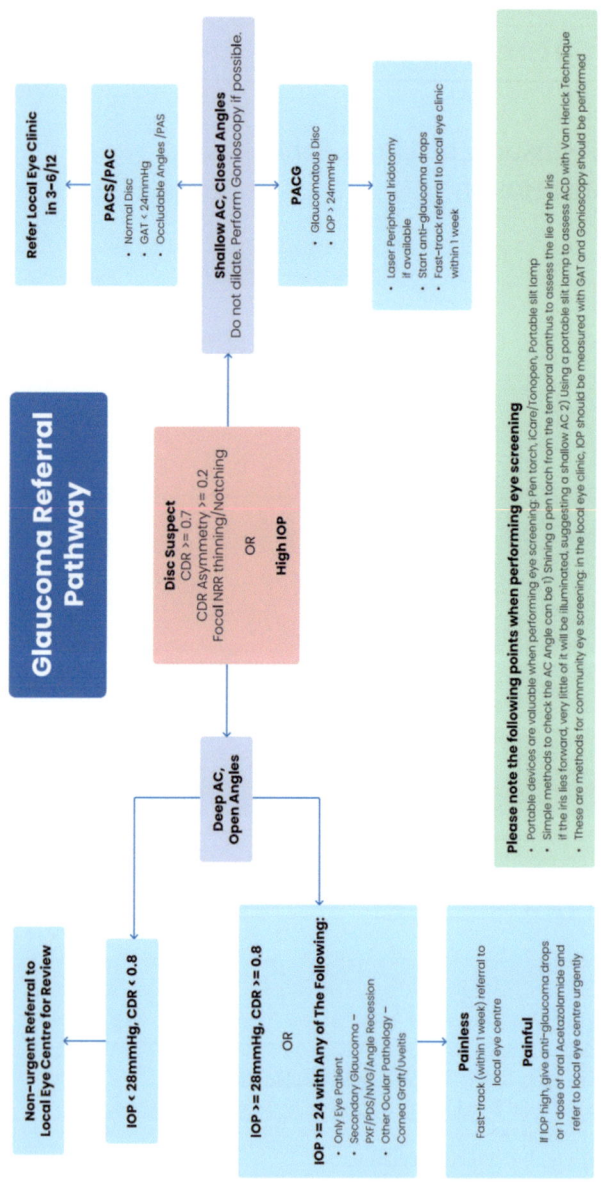

Open Access This chapter is licensed under the terms of the Creative Commons Attribution-NonCommercial-NoDerivatives 4.0 International License (http://creativecommons.org/licenses/by-nc-nd/4.0/), which permits any non-commercial use, sharing, distribution and reproduction in any medium or format, as long as you give appropriate credit to the original author(s) and the source, provide a link to the Creative Commons license and indicate if you modified the licensed material. You do not have permission under this license to share adapted material derived from this chapter or parts of it.

The images or other third party material in this chapter are included in the chapter's Creative Commons license, unless indicated otherwise in a credit line to the material. If material is not included in the chapter's Creative Commons license and your intended use is not permitted by statutory regulation or exceeds the permitted use, you will need to obtain permission directly from the copyright holder.

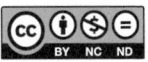

Part IV

Global Eye Health Protocols and Recommended Standards of Eye Care

Disclaimer: All text content in this part has been modified from SNEC internal guidelines, with full permission from SNEC.

Global Eye Health Guide to Improving Essential Areas of Primary and Secondary Eye Health Services

Purpose

To outline essential protocols and guidelines to adopt best practices to improve primary and secondary provision of eye health services.

These guidelines outline principles that have been written by a multidisciplinary team at the Singapore National Eye Centre and will need to be adapted, edited, and translated for the various target contexts and countries.

Hand Hygiene Protocol 51

Low Siew Ngim, Chitra Vallei, and Goh Hui Jin

Purpose

- To prevent the spread of germs from one patient to another and their environment via the hands of healthcare workers (HCWs).
- To provide guidelines to improve hand hygiene practices by HCWs to reduce tra`nsmission of pathogenic microorganisms to patients and personnel in health-care settings.

Policy

This policy applies to all staff providing care to patients.

Definition

1. Hand hygiene (HH) refers to any action of hand cleansing by HCWs, including hand washing (hand antisepsis) with soap and water, antiseptic hand wash, or alcohol-based hand rub;

L. S. Ngim · C. Vallei (✉) · G. H. Jin
Singapore National Eye Centre, Singapore Eye Research Institute, Singapore, Singapore
e-mail: low.siew.ngim@snec.com.sg; chitra.vallei@snec.com.sg; goh.hui.jin@snec.com.sg

© The Author(s) 2026
A. C S Tan et al. (eds.), *The Global Eye Health Handbook*,
https://doi.org/10.1007/978-981-96-8861-6_51

and surgical hand antisepsis (1.5–3 min hand wash with either chlorhexidine or alcohol).
2. Alcohol-based handrub refers to an alcohol-containing preparation (liquid, gel, or foam) designed for application to the hands to inactivate microorganisms and/or temporarily suppress their growth. Such preparations may contain one or more types of alcohol, other active ingredients with excipients, and humectants (ingredient(s) added to hand hygiene products to moisturise the skin).
3. Antimicrobial (medicated) soap refers to soap (detergent) containing an antiseptic agent at a concentration sufficient to inactivate microorganisms and/or temporarily suppress their growth. The detergent activity of such soaps may also dislodge transient microorganisms or other contaminants from the skin to facilitate their subsequent removal by water.
4. Antiseptic hand rubbing (or hand rubbing) refers to applying an antiseptic hand rub to reduce or inhibit the growth of microorganisms without the need for an exogenous source of water and requiring no rinsing or drying with towels or other devices.
5. Hand antisepsis refers to reducing or inhibiting the growth of microorganisms by the application of an antiseptic hand rub or by performing an antiseptic hand wash.
6. Hand care refers to actions to reduce the risk of skin damage or irritation.
7. Hand washing refers to washing hands with plain or antimicrobial soap and water.
8. PPE refers to Personal Protective Equipment.
9. Surgical hand antisepsis/surgical hand preparation refers to an antiseptic hand wash or antiseptic hand rub performed preoperatively by the surgical team to eliminate transient flora and reduce resident skin flora. Such antiseptics often have persistent antimicrobial activity.
10. *Transient flora* refers to microorganisms that colonize the superficial layers of the skin and are more amenable to removal by routine hand washing.
11. *Visibly soiled hands* refer to hands on which dirt or body fluids are readily visible.
12. *WHO* refers to World Health Organization

Procedures

Indications for Hand Hygiene

1. Wash hands with soap and water or antiseptic hand wash when visibly dirty or visibly soiled with blood or other body fluids, or after using the toilet.
2. Washing hands with non-antimicrobial liquid soap is the preferred means if exposure to potential spore-forming pathogens is strongly suspected or proven, "and gastrointestinal infection e.g. norovirus," including outbreaks of Clostridioides difficile.
3. Alcohol-based hand rub is recommended as the preferred mode for routine hand antisepsis in all other clinical situations if hands are not visibly soiled. Alcohol-based handrub is to be used on dry hands. Alcohols have excellent in vitro germicidal activity against Gram-positive and Gram-negative vegetative bacteria (including multi-drug resistant pathogens such as MRSA & VRE), Mycobacterium tuberculosis, and a wide variety of fungi. However, they have virtually no activity against bacterial spores or protozoan cysts and very poor activity against some non-enveloped (non-lipophilic) viruses.
4. Perform hand hygiene if moving from a contaminated body site to another body site during care of the same patient, after contact with inanimate surfaces and objects (including medical equipment) in the immediate vicinity of the patient, and after removing sterile or non-sterile gloves.
5. A religious bangle should be removed up the forearm during hand hygiene and secured during patient activities.
6. Remove all jewellery (rings including single flat ring or bands, bracelets or wrist watches) before entering the operating theatre or performing aseptic procedures.
7. Cover any abrasion or cuts on the hand with occlusive dressing before performing HH.
8. Soap and alcohol-based hand rub should not be used together at the same time.

Specific Indications for Hand Hygiene Based on the WHO 5 Moments

1. Moment 1: Before touching patient.
2. Moment 2: Before performing clean/aseptic procedure (i.e. before handling an invasive device for patient care, regardless of whether or not gloves are used [including before donning PPE])
3. Moment 3: After body fluid exposure risk (i.e. contact with body fluids or excretions, mucous membranes, non-intact skin, or wound dressing [including after removing PPE])
4. Moment 4: After touching patient
5. Moment 5: After touching patient surroundings

Hand Hygiene (HH) Techniques

Routine Hand Hygiene (HH)
1. Hand hygiene with alcohol-based handrub agent for 20–30 seconds is the preferred mode of hand hygiene. When hands are visibly soiled or when hands are contaminated with spore-forming bacteria without gloves protection, perform handwashing with antimicrobial soap and water at least 60 seconds.
    (a) HH technique using alcohol-based hand rub and the WHO '7-step process'
        (i) Place about 1 to 2 squirts (1.25–2.5 ml) of alcohol-based hand rub in one palm.
        (ii) Rub hands palm to palm 5 times.
        (iii) Place right palm over left dorsum with interlaced fingers and rub 5 times. Repeat with left palm over right dorsum.
        (iv) Rub 5 times palm to palm, fingers interlaced, taking care to rub sides of fingers.
        (v) With back of fingers to opposing palms with fingers interlocked, rub 5 times the knuckles.
        (vi) Perform rotational rubbing of left thumb clasped in right palm 5 times and vice versa.

(vii) Wrap left hand over right wrist using rotational movements up to mid-forearm 5 times, and vice-versa.
(viii) Once dry, your hands are safe.
(b) HH Techniques using soap and water or antimicrobial soap solution using the WHO recommended process indicated below:
(i) Wet hands with water
(ii) Rub hands palm to palm.
(iii) Place right palm over left dorsum with interlaced fingers and rub 5 times. Repeat with left palm over right dorsum.
(iv) Rub 5 times palm to palm, fingers interlaced, taking care to rub sides of fingers.
(v) With back of fingers to opposing palms with fingers interlocked, rub 5 times the knuckles.
(vi) Perform rotational rubbing of left thumb clasped in right palm 5 times; and vice versa.
(vii) Wrap left hand over right wrist using rotational movements up to mid-forearm 5 times, and vice-versa.
(viii) Rinse hands with water.
(ix) Dry hands thoroughly with a single use towel and use this towel to turn off tap. Discard towel.
(x) Your hands are now safe.

Surgical Hand Antisepsis Using Surgical Hand Preparation (Duration: 1.5–3 Min)

1. Surgical hand preparation must be used on perfectly clean, dry hands. HCWs shall adopt the surgical hand preparation technique recommended by WHO as indicated below:
   (a) Place about 4 squirts (about 5 ml) of alcohol-based hand rub into palm of left hand (using elbow of the other arm to operate the dispenser if it is not an automated dispenser).
   (b) Dip right hand fingertips into the hand rub of left palm for 5 seconds to decontaminate under the nails.

(c) Divide the right forearm into 4 planes/sections (up to the elbow).
(d) Rub each plane/section with 5 strokes (back and forth) until all the hand rub is fully evaporated; extending the rub to 5 cm above the elbow.
(e) Slightly bend your elbow to ensure all surfaces are covered.
(f) Repeat steps 1 (a) to (e) for the other hand.
(g) Place about 1 to 2 squirts (1.25 to 2.5 ml) of alcohol-based hand rub in the left palm (using the elbow of the other arm to operate the dispenser of the alcohol-based hand rub where this is not automated).
(h) Cover the whole surface of the hands up to the wrist with alcohol-based hand rub, rubbing palm against palm in a rotating movement.
(i) Rub the back of the left hand including the wrist, moving the right palm back and forth; and vice versa.
(j) Rub palm against palm with fingers interlaced, with back-and-forth movement.
(k) Rub the back of fingers of one hand by holding them in the palm of the other hand with a sideways back and forth movement; repeat with the other hand.
(l) Rub the thumb of the left hand by rotating it in the clasped palm of the right hand, and vice versa.
(m) Allow hands to dry before donning PPE.
2. Repeat the sequence (for each of the HH steps) according to the number of times corresponding to the total duration recommended by the manufacturer of the surgical antisepsis preparation with an alcohol-based hand rub.
3. Remove gloves after each procedure. Clean hands with alcohol-based hand rub or wash with antimicrobial liquid soap and water if residual talc or blood/body fluid is present.
4. Surgical hand antisepsis may also be done using same steps in 1 with surgical hand scrub agent.

Other Aspects of Hand Hygiene (HH)

1. Alcohol-based hand rubs with optimal antimicrobial efficacy usually contain 75% to 85% ethanol, isopropanol, or n-propa-

nol, or a combination of these products. The WHO recommended formulations contain either 75% v/v isopropanol, or 80% v/v ethanol. EN 1500 is to be complied with for general hand hygiene products; and EN 12791 for surgical hand hygiene products.
2. Do not refill a partially empty soap dispenser with liquid soap. This practice of 'topping up' can lead to bacterial contamination.
3. Maintain good skin care to minimize the occurrence of irritant contact dermatitis associated with hand hygiene.
4. Apply hand lotions or creams during breaks or after work to moisturize hands regularly.
5. Do not use personal hand creams at work as it may counteract the antiseptic properties in the antiseptic preparation.
6. Avoid washing hands with soap and water immediately before and after using alcohol-based hand rub as a routine.
7. Avoid donning gloves when hands are still wet with alcohol-based hand rub as this promotes bacterial growth.
8. Keep natural fingernail tips <2 mm long and pay attention to them when washing hands as microbes on hands come from beneath the fingernails.
9. Head of Department / manager or supervisor in-charge should reassign staff to non-direct patient contact tasks in situation where hand hygiene is impeded due to hand injury or other similar factors that prevent staff from being able to practise hand hygiene during clinical care (e.g. staff require hand or finger splint at all time for recovery).

Indication for Use of Gloves

1. Wear gloves when in contact with blood and other potentially infectious material.
2. Remove gloves immediately after caring for a patient to prevent HCW contamination and further transmission and dissemination of microorganisms.
3. Discard gloves appropriately immediately after use.
4. Do not wear the same pair of gloves for the care of more than one patient.

5. Change gloves in between caring for different patients or between procedures for contaminated and clean-body sites for the same patient.
6. Do not wash gloves, decontaminate, or reprocess gloves for any reuse purpose.
7. HH is required regardless of whether gloves are used or changed as hands can be contaminated by small, undetected holes in the gloves and/or during glove removal.

Bare Below Elbow Policy

1. Each institution should have Bare Below Elbow policy providing guidance to staff working at patient-fronting areas on measures to ensure effective hand hygiene.
2. Nail polish, artificial fingernails or extenders, ring, jewellery, or wristwatch are not to be worn when having direct contact with patients during care delivery.
3. Bracelets, wrist watches and rings with stones or ridges must not be worn when performing clinical care activities.
    (i) A single flat ring or band may be worn but must not interfere with effective hand hygiene practice.
    (ii) Metal bangles that are worn for religious reasons may be worn but these must be pushed up towards elbow when performing clinical care activities. Prior to an aseptic procedure, the bangle is to be removed for proper surgical hand hygiene to be done effectively.
    (iii) Sleeves must be short or rolled securely up to the elbows for effective hand hygiene.
    (iv) Long sleeves that are worn for religious reasons must be rolled up towards elbow when performing clinical care activities. Prior to an aseptic procedure, jackets must be removed for effective hand hygiene. Refer to the Guidelines on the wearing of tudung for Muslim Employees.
4. Any breached skin or non-intact skin (cuts, dermatitis, or abrasion) must be covered with a waterproof film dressing. Staff with dermatitis should seek medical consultation and evaluation.

5. Scarves or other accessories that are hanging and flowing are not to be worn at the clinical areas.
6. Tudung may be worn by Muslim staff when its use will not compromise staff or patient safety. Refer to the Guidelines on the wearing of tudung for Muslim Employees.

> **GEH Perspectives**
> 1. Hand hygiene before and after attending to patients to prevent cross infection.
> 2. Hand hygiene before and after performing a procedure.
> 3. Remember to wash your hands with soap and water if it is visibly soiled.

Open Access This chapter is licensed under the terms of the Creative Commons Attribution-NonCommercial-NoDerivatives 4.0 International License (http://creativecommons.org/licenses/by-nc-nd/4.0/), which permits any noncommercial use, sharing, distribution and reproduction in any medium or format, as long as you give appropriate credit to the original author(s) and the source, provide a link to the Creative Commons license and indicate if you modified the licensed material. You do not have permission under this license to share adapted material derived from this chapter or parts of it.

The images or other third party material in this chapter are included in the chapter's Creative Commons license, unless indicated otherwise in a credit line to the material. If material is not included in the chapter's Creative Commons license and your intended use is not permitted by statutory regulation or exceeds the permitted use, you will need to obtain permission directly from the copyright holder.

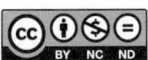

For Nurses   52

Low Siew Ngim, Chitra Vallei, and Goh Hui Jin

Aseptic Techniques

Purpose

- To establish specific guidelines for perioperative personnel to adhere closely to the principles of aseptic technique.

Policy

- Aseptic technique is a set of specific practices performed by trained perioperative staff to protect the patient from post-surgical infection. The practice and maintaining of asepsis, the absence of pathogenic organisms during surgical procedures, requires vigilance compliances in aseptic technique from all perioperative staff.

L. S. Ngim · C. Vallei (✉) · G. H. Jin
Singapore National Eye Centre, Singapore Eye Research Institute, Singapore, Singapore
e-mail: low.siew.ngim@snec.com.sg; chitra.vallei@snec.com.sg; goh.hui.jin@snec.com.sg

Definition

1. OTT refers to Operating Theatre Technician
2. Scrubbed Personnel refers to Surgeons, Assistant, and Nurses.
3. Circulating Personnel refers to Anaesthetist, Technicians, and Nurses.

Procedure

Preparation of Surgical Team

- Personnel with acute infections, such as upper respiratory tract infection should not assist in surgical procedures.
- Staff with cuts, burns, or skin lesions should not participate in the surgical procedure or handle sterile supplies.
- Fingernails must be clean and short and free from polish. Artificial nails are not permitted.
- Jewellery should be limited to one pair of stud earrings.
- Wristwatches must not be worn by staff with direct patient contact and must be removed during hand hygiene.
- Personnel entering the operating suite are required to change into clean surgical suit attire.
- Hair and facial hair must be covered completely with a disposable cap or a head-cover as hair harbours resident and transient flora.
- Disposable cap or hood should be donned before the scrub suit to avoid contamination of the suit. Caps/hoods must be removed before leaving the department.
- Surgical masks should cover the nose and mouth completely, stretching over the chin and fitting snugly over the face.
- The surface of the mask must not be handled except for the ties/loops when putting on or taking off.
- Change and dispose of the surgical mask into clinical waste immediately every 4 h or if the mask becomes moist.
- Hand hygiene must be performed before and after removal of mask.

- Hand hygiene must be carried out or alcohol rub applied correctly after each episode of patient care and before entering or leaving the department.
- Footwear must provide support and protection for the feet. It should be washable and should be washed if it becomes soiled.

General Considerations

- Sterile trolley cover should be used to establish a sterile field. The nurse must ensure that all instruments/sets introduced onto the sterile field are sterile according to the different sterilisation methods.
- Chemical indicators placed within and at the outer surface of any steam- or dry heat-sterilized item OR pouches used to contain any steam or dry heat sterilized items should change colour according to the manufacturer's recommendation to indicate that the complete cycle and parameters are met to ensure sterility.
- All Items introduced to a sterile field should be opened, dispensed, and transferred by methods that maintain sterility and integrity.
- Tables draped with sterile drapes are sterile only at table level. Items that fall below the level of the sterile field are not brought back onto the sterile field.
- Scrub personnel must not contact the edge of the instrument trolley but push it by placing the palms on top of the trolley.
- Non-sterile items should not cross over a sterile field.
- The edges of containers enclosing sterile items are not considered sterile once the container is opened.
- If there is any doubt as to the sterility of an item or surface, it is considered contaminated.

Creating a Sterile Surgical Field

Before Surgery
- Set up sterile procedure trolley just before the surgical procedure. Clean the surface of the trolley with a piece of alcohol wipe. Ensure trolley is dry and clean before laying out the sterile drape.

- It is the responsibility of the scrub nurse to check the integrity of the package, expiry date, and the appearance and colour of chemical steriliser indicating tape, processed pouch indicator strips, and process indicators outside and/or within the instruments/sets before using the instruments for preparation.
- Always face the area of sterile field during preparation. Do not turn your back to face the sterile area.
- Only the top of the sterile drape is considered sterile, the edges and sides extending below are considered unsterile. Scrub personnel must not contact the edge of the instrument trolley but push it by placing the palms on top of the trolley.
- Set sterile receptacles near the edge of the sterile tables to allow circulating nurse to dispense solutions slowly to avoid splashing.

During Surgery
- Boundaries between sterile and unsterile areas must be carefully evaluated.
    (a) The unsterile margin of the draped trolley begins at the table edge.
    (b) A one-inch safety margin is considered standard on package wrappers.
    (c) The inner edge of the heat seal package is considered the sterile boundary on peel-back packages.
- Scrubbed personnel must not lean against a non-sterile surface. Scrub personnel pass each other front-to-front or back-to-back at a 360 degree turn as the back of the gown is considered unsterile.
- Sterile instruments should not be handled across the back of other scrubbed personnel.
- Secure cords and tubing on the sterile field with a non-perforating device that will not cause puncture holes on the drapes.
- When adjusting the operating light, circulating personnel must avoid contaminating the sterile field by maintaining a safe boundary distance.
- Maintain instrument as clean as possible by removing blood and debris with a moist swab to prevent organic debris from entering the surgical site.

Draping a Non-sterile Table with Sterile Drape
- Cuff the sterile drape over gloved hands to avoid contamination of the sterile gloves.
- Cover the near side of non-sterile surface first.
- Place drape over the back of the table after the ends of the drape are unfolded over the sides of the table. Do not lift the side of the drape to the table level again. The sides of the table are considered not sterile.

Draping of Patient
1. Draping is a procedure to cover the patient and the surrounding areas with a sterile barrier to create and maintain an adequate sterile field during a surgical procedure. An effective barrier eliminates or minimises passage of pathogens between sterile and non-sterile areas.
    - Select appropriate drapes with the required specification for the different types of surgical procedures.
    - Handle drapes gently to minimise rapid stirring of air current such as dust and lint.
    - Support folded drapes with both hands and stand away from the operating table.
    - Drapes should be held higher than the operating table, avoiding the operating lights.
    - Apply drapes from the prepped operative site and extend to the periphery area.
    - Drape should not be readjusted, as a shift of the positioned drape compromises the sterility of the surgical field. The sides of the drape are considered non-sterile. An item that extends beyond the sterile boundary shall consider as contaminated.
    - Cover wet or drape with small hole with another sterile drape to prevent the migration of pathogen through the defect area.

> **GEH Perspectives**
> 1. Good aseptic technique is key to preventing post-surgical infection.
> 2. Asepsis starts with good personal hygiene.
> 3. Check the integrity of items before introducing them to the sterile field.

Eye Wash and Irrigation Procedures

Purpose

- To maintain cleanliness of the eye.
- To reduce patient's discomfort.
- To minimize potential eye infection.

Policy

- To provide a clear procedure for eye wash and irrigation pre-operatively before surgical procedures

Definition

- Eye wash and irrigation are administered as a pre-operative preparation to clean the lid and to flush away secretions and particulate matter from the eye before an intra ocular surgical procedure.

Procedure

Preparatory Phase
1. Prepare the appropriate requisites:
    - Disposable Sterile Dressing Set
    - Normal Saline 0.9% for Irrigation

- Povidone Iodine Solution 10%
- Eye Medication (Minims Tropicamide 1%, Minims Tetracine 0.5%)
- Disposable Gloves x 1 no
- Sterile Swab Sticks—1 packet
2. Introduce self to patient.
3. Identify patient against medical record using at least 2 identifiers, ensure no allergy against ordered medication:
   - Patient Name
   - Patient Identification Number/Address/Date of Birth
4. Identify site of eye for irrigation with patient.
5. Explain purpose and procedure.
6. Lie patient in a recumbent position with the head supported on a pillow.

Performance Phase
1. Perform hand rub and examine the operating eye for:
   - Lids—check for presence of discharge and oedema
   - Conjunctiva—check for infection or chemosis
   - Pupil—check the pupil size according to the type of operation.
2. Perform hand rub and open dressing set.
3. Swabs preparation:
   - Moist swabs with normal saline.
   - Moist swabs and swab sticks with Povidone Iodine 10%
4. Open eye drops as prescribed.
5. Perform hand rub and don the disposable glove.
6. Request patient to close both eyes.
7. Clean the operated eye with normal saline swab from inner canthus towards the outer canthus.
8. Request patient to open both eyes.
9. When cleaning the lower lid, request patient to look upwards and gently pull the lower lid downward. Clean the eye lid along the lower lid margin. Next clean the upper lid area.
10. To clean the upper lid, request patient to look downwards. Pull the upper lid gently upward and clean the eye lid as Step 9

11. Assist patient to turn his/her head to one side and place a receptacle beneath the eye.
12. Use the palm of your hand to support the edge of the receptacle.
13. Inform patient of cold Normal Saline irrigation and seek patient co-operation to open both eyes.
14. Hold patient's eyelid apart using your first and second fingers against the orbital ridge followed by eye irrigation.
15. Instil eye medication as ordered. Observe the protocol on eye drops.
16. Alert patient on the stingy effects of the eye drops.
17. Use the Iodine coated swab stick to apply on the lower lash line. Request patient to look up and gently expose the lower lash line by everting lower lid downwards. Carefully apply from inner canthus towards outer.
18. Repeat Step 17 with the upper lash line. Request patient to look down and gently expose the upper lash line by everting upper lid upwards. Carefully apply from inner canthus towards outer.
19. With the patient's eyes remaining closed, saturate the cotton swab in Povidone Iodine 10% and coat the eyelid in the following sequences:
    - On the eyelashes, from the inner canthus x 1st swab.
    - On the upper eyelid, extending above the brow area x 2nd swab.
    - On the lower eyelid, up to the orbital rim x 3rd swab.
20. Exercise care to prevent undiluted Povidone Iodine 10% from entering the eye.
21. Remind patient to keep the eyes closed for a few seconds.
22. Inform patient of the completion of eye toilet. Refer to Annexes. Request patient to remain on the trolley and ask for assistance if necessary.

Follow-Up Phase

1. Dispose soiled consumables and gloves.
2. Perform hand wash.

> **GEH Perspectives:**
> 1. Check patient's eyes for any abnormalities, before performing Eye Wash.
> 2. Report any abnormal findings to the Doctor before performing the Eye Wash, as procedure maybe cancelled.
> 3. Flush the eye generously with normal saline, to ensure all secretions and particles are flushed away.

Eye Dressing

Purpose

- To maintain cleanliness of the eye.
- To reduce patient's discomfort
- To minimize potential eye infection

Policy

- To establish standard procedure for Eye Dressing.

Definition

- Eye Dressing, also known as Eye Toilet, is performed for the removal of any debris that may have accumulated on the eye lashes, to reduce infection and to prepare the eye for instillation of medication or to maintain eye comfort.

Procedure

Preparatory Phase
1. Obtain appropriate requisites:
   - Disposable Dressing Set
   - Disposable Gloves

- Normal Saline for Irrigation
- Micropore Tape
- Eye Shield/Pad
- Eye Medication (indicate date of opening)
- Tissue paper
- Mirror (if necessary)
- Pen Torch
- Waste Bag
- Relevant Educational Pamphlet

2. Check Doctor's order for eye dressing and eye medication in patient's medical records.
3. Introduce self to patient.
4. Identify patient against medical records, using at least 2 identifiers:
   - Patient Name
   - Patient Identification Number/Address/Date of Birth
5. Check that patient is not allergic to the drugs prescribed by verifying with the medical records and by asking the patient.
6. Check post-op instructions and eye medication.
7. Explain purpose and procedure to patient.
8. Position patient comfortably in a sitting position, with the head tilted slightly backwards OR lie patient in a recumbent position, with head supported on a pillow.
9. Provide a mirror for patient to view the procedure if necessary.

Performance Phase

1. Perform hand wash and don gloves.
2. Remove eye shield or eye pad if present.
3. Observe any discharges on the eye pad before discarding into the waste bag.
4. Wash and dry eye shield and place the clean eye shield-lower case at a corner inside the dressing set.
5. Remove and discard gloves.
6. Wash and dry hands before cleaning the eye.
7. Don a new pair of gloves.
8. Moist swabs with normal saline and squeeze out excess saline solution into waste bag.
9. Remove any discharges if present, before commencing eye dressing.

10. Clean the operated eye, using the swab once only, in the following manner:
    - Ask patient to close both eyes.
    - Wipe the surface area of the operated eye from the inner canthus to the outer canthus.
    - Cleaning the lower lid:
        - Ask patient to look upwards.
        - Gently pull the lower lid downwards.
        - Clean along the lower lid margin.
        - Clean the lower lid area.
    - Cleaning the upper Lid
        - Ask patient to look downwards.
        - Gently pull the upper lid upwards.
        - Clean along the upper lid margin.
        - Clean the upper lid area.
11. Remove and discharge gloves.
12. Perform hand wash.
13. Examine the operated eye with a pen torch before instillation of eye drops or application of Ointment:
    - Lids—Check for presence of discharges, oedema, and redness.
    - Conjunctiva—Check for redness or chemosis.
    - Wound Section—Check surgical wound site for presence of haematoma, loose sutures, or infection.
14. Perform hand rub.
15. Instil or apply the prescribed eye drops/ointment.
16. Apply eye pad/eye shield if necessary and secure with micropore tape.
17. If eye shield is not used, return to patient in a ziploc bag.
18. Perform hand rub.

Follow-Up Phase

1. Obtain verbal feedback from patient/caregiver to affirm their ability in performing eye dressing.
2. Document procedure performed onto the medical records.
3. Record abnormalities, if present, onto the medical records and inform the attending Doctor.

4. Dispose soiled consumables and disinfect trolley.
5. Perform hand wash.

> **GEH Perspectives**
> 1. Maintain sterility to prevent infection.
> 2. Monitor for complications of post-surgery.
> 3. Emphasize on compliance to post-op medication and follow-up visit.
> 4. Use protective shields or goggles to prevent accidental trauma.

Instillation of Eyedrops and Application of Eye Ointment

Purpose

- To perform fundus examination.
- To treat various eye conditions.
- To anaesthetize the eye.

Policy

- To establish standard procedure for instillation of eyedrops and application of eye ointment.

Definition

- Eyedrop instillation and eye ointment application are effective methods of drug delivery into a patient's eye. Both eyedrops and ointments are routinely administered in the clinics and by the patients at home.

Procedure

Preparatory Phase
1. Obtain appropriate requisites:
   - Lint Squares
   - Eye medication
   - Pen torch
   - Waste bag
2. Check doctor's order of eye medication from the medical record.
3. Introduce self to patient.
4. Identify patient against patient medical records, using at least 2 identifiers:
   - Patient's name
   - Patient's identification number/Address/Date of birth
5. Check that patient is not allergic to the drugs prescribed by verifying with the patient's medical record and by asking the patient.
6. Explain purpose and procedure to patient and any possible side effects e.g. blurring of near vision, stinging sensation, etc.
7. Position patient comfortably in a sitting/lying position with the head tilted slightly backwards.

Performance Phase
1. Perform hand hygiene.
2. Remove eye shield or eye pad if present.
3. Ask patient to look upwards.
4. Gently pull the lower lid downwards to expose the lower fornix.
5. With the other hand, hold the eyedrop bottle about 2.5 cm from the eye and instil 1 or 2 drops into the centre of the lower fornix.
6. When applying ointment, squeeze some away before applying it onto the inside of the lower fornix, beginning at the inner canthus, and moving outwards. The lid may be massaged gently in such a way as Instruct patient to blink the eye a few times to distribute the drug over the eyeball.

7. The tip of the eyedrop bottle or ointment tube should not touch the eyelashes or lid during instillation/application.
8. Ask patient to close the eye gently to prevent squeezing out the eye medication.
9. Wipe off excess fluid from the eye with the lint squares.
10. Apply eye pad/eye shield if necessary and secure with micropore tape.
11. Inform patient of the possible side effects of the eye medication such as some stinging sensation or blurring of vision.
12. Perform hand hygiene.

Follow-Up Phase
1. Affirm with patient/caregiver on their ability to perform instillation of eyedrops/application of eye ointment.
2. Document procedure performed into the medical record.

> **GEH Perspectives**
> 1. Ensure patient identification and medication verification.
> 2. Wash hands and use gloves to prevent contamination.
> 3. Tilt patient's head to ensure eye drop is instilled on to the lower fornix.
> 4. Instruct patient to blink eye a few times following application of ointment to spread the ointment across the eye.
> 5. Document administration and patient response.

Administration of Medication

Purpose

- To ensure the safe administration and monitoring of medication.

Policy

- This policy sets out guidelines for nurses to administer medication prescribed by the doctor to patients under their care.

Definition

1. Administration of medication consists of:
   - Instillation of eyedrops/Application of eye ointment
   - Administering of oral medication
   - Administration of intradermal injection
   - Administration of subcutaneous injection
   - Administration of intramuscular injection
   - Administration of intravenous therapy
   - Assisting in insertion of peripheral intravenous line
   - Insertion of rectal suppository

Guidelines

1. Instillation of eyedrops/Application of eye ointment/Insertion of rectal suppository—performed by trained personnel.
2. Administering of oral Medication/intradermal injection/subcutaneous injection/intramuscular injection/intravenous therapy—performed only by trained personnel.
3. Check the doctor's written order of the medication in the patient's medical record. All medication orders must be signed and dated by the doctor.
4. Medication orders should be prescribed by the attending doctor. Any ambiguous medication order should be clarified with the doctor.
5. Look-alike and sound-alike drugs must be appropriately segregated and identified.
6. Accept verbal orders over telephone in emergency situations only. Upon receipt of the verbal order, the nurse will:

- Read back the patient's name, the name of the drug, the dose, the route of administration, the frequency and duration for which the drug is to be administered.
- Obtain confirmation from the individual who gave the order that the read back order is correct.

7. When Reading Back the order:
   - Spell out the name of the drug(s) ordered using alphabet recognition aids e.g. 'A' for America, 'B' for Bangkok, 'C' China.
   - Numbers should be broken down; for example '15' should be stated as 'one five' to avoid confusion with the number 50.
   - Do not use abbreviations; for example '1 tab tid' should be read back as 'One tablet three times daily'.
8. The person who receives the order should document, date, and note the time of the order.
9. Before administering medication, always check the expiry date of the drug and staff must verify the 8 Rs (Rights):
   - The *Right* Patient
   - The *Right* Medication
   - The *Right* Dosage
   - The *Right* Route
   - The *Right* Time and Frequency
   - The *Right* Speed of Injection
   - The *Right* Diluent
   - The *Right* Site
10. For administration of oral medication/intradermal injection/subcutaneous injection/intramuscular injection/intravenous therapy/insertion of rectal suppository, perform a double check system.
11. Check that patient is not allergic to the drug prescribed by verifying with the medical record/and by asking the patient.
12. Explain the procedure and advise the patient on the medications.
    - Its purpose and relevance to the patient's condition
    - Possible side effects e.g. blurring of vision, stinging sensation, etc.

13. Monitor the patient's response to the medication in the medical record and contact the doctor immediately if patient develops a reaction to the drug.
14. Document in the patient's medical record that the drug has been administered.
15. Ensure that patient is comfortable and has no adverse drug reactions before discharging patient home.

> **GEH Perspectives**
> 1. Verify medication orders and patient allergies.
> 2. Comply to the 8 Rights of medication.
> 3. Check for drug allergy prior to administration of medication.
> 4. Educate patient on medication purpose, dosage, and potential side effects.

Assisting in Fundus Angiography

Policy

- To establish standard procedure for fundus angiography.

Purpose

- To ensure that the procedure for fundus angiography is carried out safely.
- To study the blood flow of the innermost layers of the eye, the retina and choroid and identify blood vessels that are leaking or damaged.

Definition

1. FA refers to fundus angiography, which is a diagnostic procedure that uses special dye(s) and a special camera to take photographs of the blood vessels inside of the eye.

2. FFA refers to fundus fluorescein angiography.
3. ICG refers to indocyanine green.
4. IV refers to Intravenous.

Procedure

Preparatory Phase

1. Obtain appropriate requisites:
   - Injection dyes
     - Injection sodium fluorescein 10%
     - Injection indocyanine green 25 mg (ICG)
   - Sterile water for Injection
   - Medication
     - Tablet Loratadine 10 mg (Anti-Histamine)
     - Tablet Maxolon 10 mg (Anti-Emetic)
   - Dilating Eyedrops
     - Gutt Tropicamide 1%
     - Gutt Phenylephrine 2.5% (if required)
   - Tray containing
     - Disposable syringe of required size—3cc/5cc/10cc
     - Disposable needle of required size—19G

   - IV cannula 22G
   - Alcohol swab sachets
   - Tegaderm
   - Elastoplast strip
   - Sharp disposal container
   - Blood pressure monitoring device
   - Resuscitation trolley on standby
2. Check doctor's written order for the type of drugs to be used for the procedure in patient's medical.
3. Introduce self to patient.
4. Identify patient against medical record using at least 2 identifiers:
   - Patient name
   - Patient identification number/Address/Date of Birth
5. Explain charges to patient.

6. Prepare prescribed medication and perform a double check system.
7. Observe the guidelines on Administration of Medication.
8. Check that the patient is not allergic to the drugs prescribed by verifying with the medical record and by asking the patient. For ICG, check if patient has had an allergic reaction to iodine, iodine-related dye or shellfish.
9. Ensure that the doctor explains to patient the purpose and any side effects and obtains consent from patient.
10. Refer to 'Fundus Angiography FAQs and Patient Consent Form' frequently asked questions and consent form, at Annex.

Performance Phase
1. Perform hand wash/hand rub.
2. Ensure visual acuity and intraocular pressure is done prior to FFA.
3. Dilate both pupils fully.
4. Check and record patient's vital signs:
   - Blood pressure
   - Pulse rate
5. Serve prescribed medications:
   - Tablet Loratadine 10 mg to relief allergies.
   - Tablet Maxolon 10 mg to prevent vomiting.
6. Hand over the prepared FA drugs to the Ophthalmic Imaging Specialists, who will assist the doctor/nurse/trained personnel in the administration of drugs for FA. Time out is to be done by the attending doctor and nurse.
7. Position patient comfortably in front of the camera with chin and forehead resting firmly on the frame.
8. Photographs of the fundus are taken before the injection of the drugs by the Ophthalmic Imaging Specialist.
9. The doctor/nurse will perform the following:
   - Insert the IV cannula into the patient's vein.
   - Inject the drugs via the IV cannula.
   - A series of photographs of the fundus are taken once the drug has been injected into the eye for up to 30 min. These pictures are known as angiograms.

10. Observe patient's comfort and any allergic reactions throughout the procedure.
11. Remove the IV cannula and apply elastoplast strip.
12. Clear the requisites and discard sharps into sharp disposal container.
13. Perform hand wash/hand rub.

Follow-Up Phase

1. Record the date and time of the procedure performed onto the patient's medical record.
2. Leave the IV line for about 30 min after the Angiography to observe for any reaction in case resuscitation is required.
3. Ensure that patient is comfortable.
4. Doctor to review patient and if fit for discharge, to ensure that the IV cannula is removed before discharging patient home.
5. Advise and issue information on Post-Fundus Angiography procedure and inform patient to drink plenty of water to flush the fluorescein or ICG dye from the body. Refer to Annex—Fundus Angiography Post-investigation Care and Advice
6. Advise patient on the follow-up review date.

GEH Perspectives
1. Ensure patient understanding of procedure and consent.
2. Maintain patient comfort and positioning.
3. Monitor patient's vital signs and reaction to the injected dye.

Administration of Intravitreal Therapy Injection

Purpose

1. To establish the roles and responsibilities of the trained ophthalmic personnel administering the IVT injections.

2. To treat posterior segment diseases via intravitreal injection of:
    - Steroids e.g. Triamcinolone Acetonide
    - Anti-VEGF e.g. Bevacizumab, Ranibizumab, Aflibercept, Faricimab

Policy

- Only ophthalmic personnel who had been certified competent in administering IVT injection are allowed to perform this procedure. The administration of intravitreal injections requires specialized training of ophthalmic personnel and various ophthalmic practices are encouraged to perform rigorous training, upskilling, and auditing for the quality and safety of their intravitreal injections administered.

Definition

1. IVT refers to Intravitreal Therapy.
2. IOP refers to Intra-Ocular Pressure.
3. Anti-VEGF refers to Anti-Vascular Endothelial Growth Factor.

Procedure

Preparatory Phase
1. Obtain appropriate requisites:
   - Intravitreal Set
     – IVT disposable set or equivalent autoclaved sterile set
   - Povidone Iodine 10% to clean the patient's eyelids.
   - Gutt/Minims Tetracaine 1% (Topical Anaesthetic drop).
   - Gutt/Minims Povidone Iodine 5%
   - Prescribed Drugs
     – Triamcinolone Acetonide
     – Bevacizumab
     – Ranzibizumab

- Aflibercept
- Dexamethasone implant (Ozurdex)
- Faricimab
- Disposable Syringe of required size—1cc
- Disposable Needle of required size—19G/27G/30G
- Alcohol swab sachets
- Sterile Gloves
- Surgical Mask
- Gauze
- Sharp Disposal Container
2. Ensure that eye evaluation tests are done prior to IVT and the results documented:
    - Non-Contact Intraocular Pressure
3. Check doctor's written order of medication in patient's medical record. Nurse must trigger and document the order series of IVT drug in the medical record.
4. Observe the Guidelines on Administration of Medication.
5. Prepare prescribed medication and perform a double check system, either by a Dr and trained ophthalmic personnel or by two trained ophthalmic personnel.
6. Introduce self to patient.
7. Identify patient against medical record using at least 2 identifiers:
    - Patient Name
    - Patient Identification Number/Address/Date of Birth
8. Indicate the site for the procedure with the appropriate site marking sticker on patient's forehead.
    - For Right side—denoted by 'RIGHT'.
    - For Left side—denoted by 'LEFT'.
9. Check that patient is not allergic to the drug prescribed by verifying with the medical record and by asking the patient.
10. Ensure that the doctor explains to patient the purpose and relevance of medication and any side effects and obtains consent from patient.
11. Position patient comfortably in a semi-recumbent position.

Performance Phase

1. Perform hand wash.
2. Use sterile gloves and masks.
3. Instil 2–4 drops of topical anaesthetic (Gutt/Minims Tetracaine 1%) into the lower fornix.
4. The nurse injector will perform the following:
   - Clean the eyelid, eyelashes, and skin with 10% Povidone Iodine solution.
     - Inspect for red/swollen eye lids, purulent discharge, visible crusting.
     - In the event that the patient is allergic to povidone iodine, to clean with 0.1% aqueous chlorhexidine.
   - Apply 2 drops of 5% Povidone Iodine solution to site of injection.
     - In the event that the patient is allergic to povidone iodine, to instil 0.1% aqueous chlorhexidine.
   - Apply drape over injection site.
   - Insert eyelid speculum.
   - Withdraw the dose of the drug using the 1cc syringe and 19G needle, then change to 30G needle.
   - Cotton swab stick may be used to stabilize the globe.
   - Insert needle of size 30G through the pars plana in the inferotemporal quadrant 3.5 to 4 mm posterior to the limbus.
   - Inject the drug slowly into the vitreous cavity. Rapid injection causes excessive dispersion of the drug into the vitreous cavity and can cause the needle to come off the syringe.
   - Observe the patient's comfort and any allergic reactions throughout the procedure.
   - Remove the needle carefully from the eye after the injection and apply a sterile cotton-tip applicator to the injection site to prevent reflux of both the drug and the vitreous.
   - Flush the eye with normal saline 0.9% to remove remnant iodine.
   - Cover the non-injection eye and perform visual acuity by counting finger.

- Reinforce to patient not to rub the injected eye and do not let water enter the eye for 24 h.
5. Discharge patient with post IVT education advice.
6. Remove site marking sticker from patient's forehead.
7. Continue to observe patient's comfort and any allergic reactions throughout the procedure.
8. Clear the requisites and discard sharps into sharp disposal container.
9. Perform hand wash.

Follow-Up Phase

1. Observe, record, and report patient's response to the medication (if any) into patient's medical record and inform the attending doctor.
2. Reassure patient that some blurring of vision, which is often described as seeing spots floating in the eye (floaters) is common post-injection. These floaters usually resolve after a few days or weeks.
3. Advise and issue information on post intravitreal injection to patients. Refer to Annex—Intravitreal Therapy (IVT) Post-injection Care and Advice.
4. Continue with the prescribed medication as advised by the doctor.
5. Advise patient on the follow-up review date.

GEH Perspectives
1. Complete specialised training and competency verification before administering IVT.
2. Follow strict aseptic technique.
3. Use topical anaesthesia and ensure patient comfort.
4. Monitor for IVT injection complications (e.g. bleeding, reduced or loss of vision).

Annexes

Eyelid Hygiene Advice

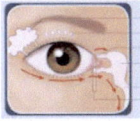

Large lacrimal gland
Accessory lacrimal gland
Lacrimal canaliculi
Lacrimal sac
Nasal lacrimal duct
Punctum

Lacrimal drainage system

Maintaining good eyelid hygiene helps to control the symptoms and severity of inflammation of the eyelids and dry eyes. Thorough eyelid cleansing will help remove debris, crust and discharges from the lid margin. You can relieve the irritation by following the steps below.

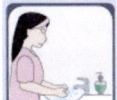

❶ Wash your hands with soap and water.

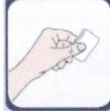

❷ Fold the cotton linen into a small rectangle.

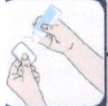
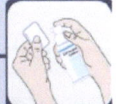

❸ Apply a small amount of eyelid cleanser on the cotton linen.

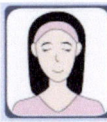

❹ Close your eyes gently. Eyelid margins will not be prominent if you squeeze your eyes.

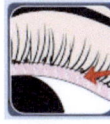

❺ Upper eyelid: Use your finger to gently lift the upper eyelid so that the margin is visible. Holding a cotton linen in another hand, scrub several times along the eyelid margin where the eye lash meets the skin.

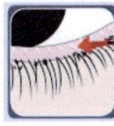

❻ Lower eyelid: Use your finger to gently pull the lower eyelid so that the margin is visible. Holding a cotton linen in another hand, scrub several times along the eyelid margin where the eye lash meets the skin.

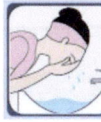

❼ Rinse under the tap water or use a damp face towel to clean away the eyelid cleanser especially at the eye lashes region.

Warm Compress

Applying warm compress can help to loosen the debris/crusts on the lashes, allowing for easier removal with the eyelid cleanser.

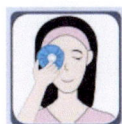

Steps:
1. Use a clean towel or cotton pad soaked in warm water.
2. Close your eyes and apply warm compress to your eyelids for 5 minutes.
3. Repeat the warm compress when necessary.

Do not use lid cleanser if:
- You are allergic to any of the ingredients listed in the product leaflet.
- Swelling of eyelids, excessive itchiness or irritation occurs after the use of the products

Images reproduced with permission and courtesy of SNEC.

Fundus Angiography FAQs and Patient Consent Form (2 pages)

FUNDUS ANGIOGRAPHY

What you should know before going for the test

What is angiography of the fundus?

Fundus angiography is a test that uses special dyes and a special camera to take photographs of the inside of the eye.

Why is this test done?

This is to study the blood flow of the innermost layers of the eye, i.e. retina and the choroid. It will identify blood vessels that are leaking or damaged. The test result will guide your doctor in the treatment of your eye condition.

Is the test an x-ray?

Only photographs are taken. No x-rays or harmful forms of radiation are involved.

How is the test performed?

This is an outpatient procedure that will take about 1 hour in total.

Eye drops are first used to dilate the pupils. The chin is placed on a chin rest with the forehead pressed forwards against the support bar.

A suitable vein is identified on the arm/hand so that the doctor can set an intravenous line for the dye to be injected.

Many photographs are taken once the dye has been injected for up to 30 minutes.

How should I prepare for the test?

You should come accompanied as your pupils will be dilated and your vision may be blurred after the test.

What dyes are used?

There are 2 dyes- fluorescein and indocyanine green (ICG).

Are there side effects?

Injection of fluorescein will lead to transient orange discolouration of the skin, tears and urine. This lasts for few hours.

Indocyanine green is related to iodine. **If you have had an allergic reaction to iodine, iodine- related dyes or shellfish, you should let us know** and the test may have to be cancelled.

Side effects occur at a rate of less than 5% of all tests. Mild side effects such as nausea and vomiting may occur. Moderate side effects such as syncope (fainting) and skin rashes can develop. These generally respond well to treatment. To reduce the effects of any allergy we will prescribe pre-procedural Loratadine 10mg and Maxolon 10mg tablets unless your doctor indicates otherwise.

Severe reactions are rare but require immediate attention if they occur. These include severe allergic reactions, shock and cardiac arrest. Emergency resuscitation will be necessary as these are potentially life-threatening.

I have read and understood the procedure and the potential side effects of fundal angiography. I agree to undergo this procedure.

Name & IC number   Signature & Date

I confirm that I have explained the nature, purpose and effect of the operation to the consenting person who acknowledged having understood it fully and signed the same in my presence.

Surgeon's Signature   Date

Name

Witness's Signature   Date

Name

Form reproduced with permission and courtesy of SNEC.

Fundus Angiography Post-investigation Care and Advice

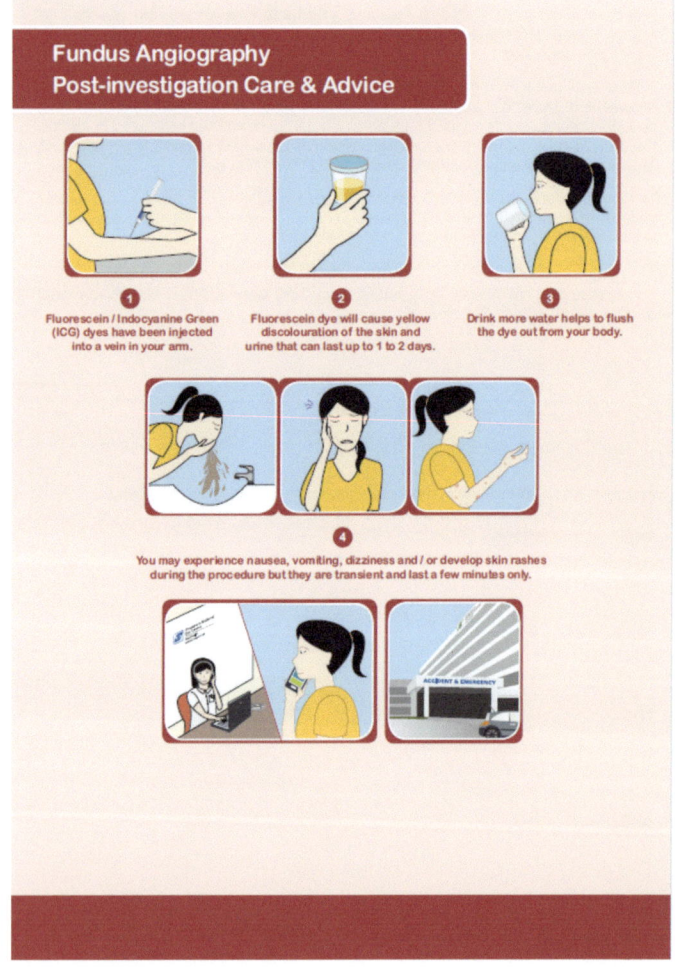

Images reproduced with permission and courtesy of SNEC.

Intravitreal Therapy (IVT) Post-injection Care and Advice

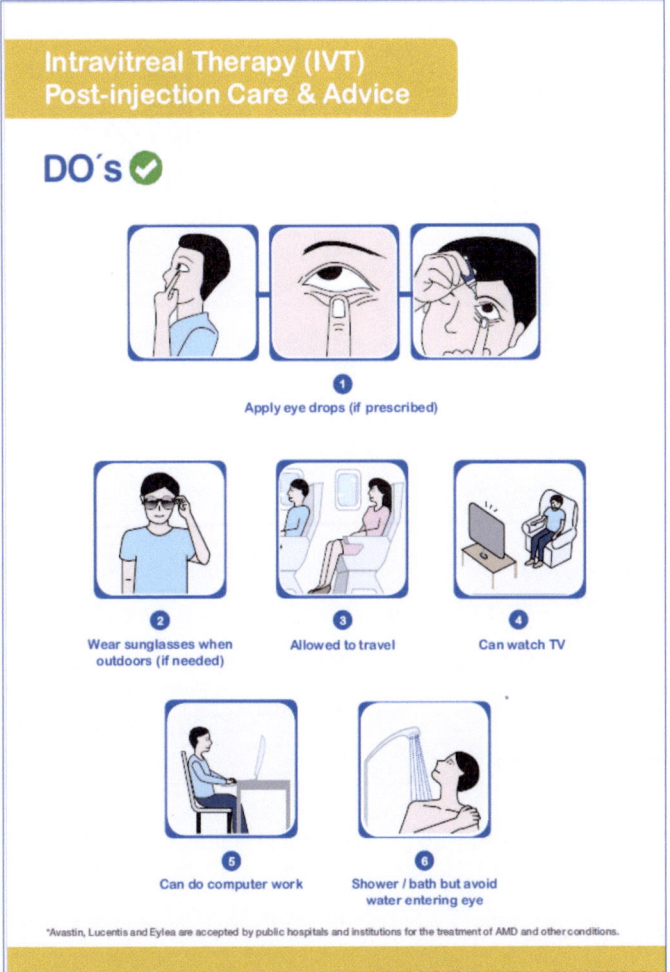

Images reproduced with permission and courtesy of SNEC.

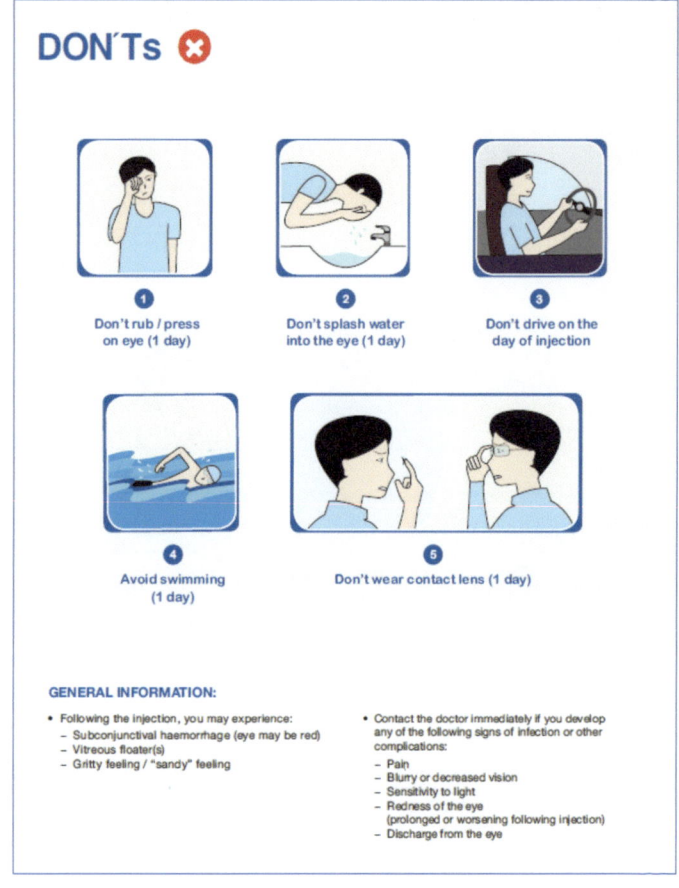

Images reproduced with permission and courtesy of SNEC.

References

Rothrock, J.C., Smith, D.A. & Mcewen, D. R. (2007), Alexander's Care of The Patient In Surgery (13th Ed.). USA: Mosby.

Association of Operating Room Nurses (AORN) Standards of Practice Maintaining a Sterile Field

Open Access This chapter is licensed under the terms of the Creative Commons Attribution-NonCommercial-NoDerivatives 4.0 International License (http://creativecommons.org/licenses/by-nc-nd/4.0/), which permits any non-commercial use, sharing, distribution and reproduction in any medium or format, as long as you give appropriate credit to the original author(s) and the source, provide a link to the Creative Commons license and indicate if you modified the licensed material. You do not have permission under this license to share adapted material derived from this chapter or parts of it.

The images or other third party material in this chapter are included in the chapter's Creative Commons license, unless indicated otherwise in a credit line to the material. If material is not included in the chapter's Creative Commons license and your intended use is not permitted by statutory regulation or exceeds the permitted use, you will need to obtain permission directly from the copyright holder.

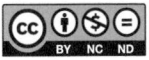

For Nurses

53

Low Siew Ngim, Chitra Vallei, and Goh Hui Jin

Laser Safety Precaution

Purpose

- To ensure that staff working with Lasers understand the 'Standard Laser Safety Precautions and Practices'.

Policy

- This policy sets out guidelines and procedures on Laser Safety Precautions.

Definition

1. LASER is an acronym for Light Amplification by Stimulated Emission of Radiation. The laser produces an intense and highly directional beam of light, which is potentially hazardous because it can burn the retina of the eye or even the skin.

L. S. Ngim · C. Vallei (✉) · G. H. Jin
Singapore National Eye Centre, Singapore Eye Research Institute, Singapore, Singapore
e-mail: low.siew.ngim@snec.com.sg; chitra.vallei@snec.com.sg; goh.hui.jin@snec.com.sg

2. Laser safety is the avoidance of laser accidents, especially those involving eye injuries.
3. Non-Ionising Radiation Irradiating apparatus refers to apparatus that were brought under legislative control (The Radiation Protection Act, 1991), such as medical ultrasound machines, lasers, etc.
4. Laser Nurse in-Charge refers to a registered nurse, or equivalent ophthalmic personnel, who oversees the day-to-day running of the Laser Centre/Room and ensures environmental safety during laser procedures.

Guidelines

1. With the 'Radiation Protection Act, 1991', Institutions will need to apply for an appropriate license to have in possession a non-ionizing apparatus to ensure the safety of the operator and users of the equipment based on their own country's legislation.
2. The Laser Nurse In-Charge will be required to:
    - Ensure Standardised Laser Precautions and Practices.
        – Environmental Safety during laser procedures.
        – Laser Machines are licensed with the appropriate Laser License.
        – Ensure that the Laser Machines are serviced regularly and are in proper working condition.
        – Proper Installation, Commissioning and Testing of any new acquired Laser Machine.
    - Keep records on the list of doctors privileged to perform laser treatment.
    - Ensure that each laser machine has a Laser Manual for easy reference.
    - Manage the day-to-day operations of the Laser Centre/Room and continually monitor safety procedures. Refer to Annex—Pre-laser Safety Checklist.
        – Perform daily checks on the laser machine cables, bulbs and switches to ensure that they are not loose or frayed.

- Maintain neatness and tidiness of the laser rooms.
    - Ensure proper handling, cleaning, and maintenance of laser lenses.
  - Orientate staff on Laser Safety Precautions in the laser environment.
  - Contact service contract provider for equipment breakdown when the need arises and follow-up on progress status of the machine.
3. Precautions to be taken to ensure Laser Safety:
   - There should be 'Laser Warning Symbol' displayed prominently on all laser room doors or Laser Panels showing 'Laser in Progress' to alert personnel not to enter the laser room.
   - Door to the laser room should be closed whenever the laser is in use.
   - Laser Safety Goggles should be made available and worn by personnel working in the laser room to prevent ocular injuries.
     - These goggles should have side shields of appropriate wavelength and adequate optical density.
     - Check eyewear for any scratches and cracks as this will lead to less protection from laser light.
   - Laser Keys should only be handled by Laser Nurse In-Charge and kept locked in a designated place when not in use. The key must not be left in the switch when the laser system is unattended.
   - Avoid placing combustible materials such as paper products, drapes, alcohol, etc. near the path of the beam as it may ignite if struck by laser beams.
   - Fire Extinguisher must be readily available at the Laser Centre/Clinic.
   - During any laser procedure in which a fire erupts, turn off the laser machine immediately and ensure patient and staff safety.

> **GEH Perspectives**
> 1. Explain procedure to patient and obtain consent.
> 2. Wear protective eyewear (laser-safe goggles).
> 3. Maintain patient stability and positioning.
> 4. Ensure laser alignment and calibration.
> 5. Follow laser safety protocols.

Assisting in YAG Posterior Capsulotomy Laser

Purpose

- To create a hole in the thickened Posterior Lens Capsule to allow light to pass through the membrane to the retina at the back of the eye and restore clear vision.

Policy

- To establish standard procedure for YAG Posterior Capsulotomy Laser.

Definition

1. Nd:YAG Laser refers to Neodynium Yttrium Aluminium Garnet Laser. It is used to correct Posterior Capsule Opacification, a complication of Cataract Surgery and for Peripheral Iridotomy in patients with Acute Angle-Closure Glaucoma.
2. PCO refers to Posterior Capsule Opacification, which is also known as 'After Cataract' or 'Secondary Membrane' that may develop gradually in some patients over several months or years after Cataract Surgery affecting the person's vision and lifestyle.

Procedure

Preparatory Phase

1. Obtain appropriate requisites:
   - Abraham Capsulotomy YAG Lens
   - Vidisic Gel (Lens Lubricant)
   - Topical Anaesthetic Drops
     - Gutt/Minims Tetracaine 1%
     - Gutt Proparacaine 0.5%
   - Dilating Eye Drops
     - Gutt Tropicamide 1%
     - Gutt Phenylephrine 2.5% (if required)
   - Laser Goggles
   - Alcohol Wipes
   - Tissue Paper
   - Waste Bag
2. Check doctor's written order to perform YAG Posterior Capsulotomy Laser in patient's medical record.
3. Introduce self to patient.
4. Identify patient against medical record using at least 2 identifiers:
   - Patient Name
   - Patient Identification Number/Address/Date of Birth
5. Indicate the site for the procedure with the appropriate site marking sticker on patient's forehead.
   - For Right side—denoted by 'RIGHT' sticker.
   - For Left side—denoted by 'LEFT' sticker.
6. Prepare prescribed medication and perform a double check system, by 2 authorised personnel.
7. Observe the Guidelines on Administration of Medication.
8. Check that the patient is not allergic to the drugs prescribed by verifying with the medical record and by asking the patient.
9. Ensure that the doctor explains to patient the purpose and any side effects and obtains consent from patient.
10. Complete the 'Pre-laser safety checklist'. Refer to Annex—Pre-laser Safety Checklist

Performance Phase

1. Perform hand wash/hand rub.
2. Prior to the Laser procedure, instil the following eye drops into patient's affected eye:
   - Gutt Tropicamide 1% to dilate the pupil.
   - Gutt Proparacaine 0.5% or Gutt/Minims Tetracaine 1% (topical anaesthetic drops) to anaesthetize the eye.
3. Wipe the essential parts of the machine that comes in contact with the patient with alcohol wipes before start of procedure.
4. Position patient comfortably in front of the Slit Lamp with chin and forehead resting firmly on the frame and strap patient's head before commencement of Laser procedure if necessary.
5. Doctor will perform the following:
   - Do site marking with skin marker.
   - Place a Laser lens on the eye to direct the Laser light into the eye.
   - Perform the Laser treatment.
6. Ensure patient's comfort after the Laser.
7. Wipe the essential parts of the machine that comes in contact with the patient with alcohol wipes after the procedure.
8. Perform hand wash/ hand rub.

Follow-Up Phase

1. Record the date and time of the YAG Laser performed onto the patient's medical record.
2. Advise and issue information on post-laser procedure to patient.
3. Continue with the prescribed medication as advised by the doctor.
4. Advise patient on the follow-up review date.
5. Refer to Annexes Laser Treatment Checklist, and Post Laser Care and Advice.

> **GEH Perspectives**
> 1. Verify correct patient, procedure, and site of procedure, ensuring informed consent has been obtained.
> 2. Ensure pupil is well dilated and maintain patient stability and positioning, using the appropriate laser protection goggles for assistants.
> 3. Monitor laser settings and alignment and proper servicing of machine.
> 4. Ensure the patient understands possible side-effects and symptoms of complications.

Assisting in Laser Peripheral Iridotomy (PI)

Purpose

- To decrease the IOP in patients with narrow angle glaucoma or angle-closure glaucoma.

Policy

- To establish standard procedure for Laser Peripheral Iridotomy (PI).

Definition

1. Laser PI refers to Laser Peripheral Iridotomy, which is the application of a laser beam through the iris without removal of the iris tissue. It enhances the drainage passage blocked by a portion of the iris.
2. IOP refers to Intra-Ocular Pressure, which is pressure caused by the fluid inside the eye that helps maintain the shape of the eye.

Procedure

Preparatory Phase

1. Obtain appropriate requisites:
   - Abraham Iridectomy (Argon) Lens
   - Abraham Iridectomy (YAG) Lens
   - Gutt Brominidine if required (Glaucoma Eye drop)
   - Vidisic Gel (Lens Lubricant)
   - Topical Anaesthetic Drops
     - Gutt/Minims Tetracaine 1%
     - Gutt Proparacaine 0.5%
   - Miotics (Constricting) Eye Drops
     - Gutt Pilocarpine 2%
   - Laser Goggles
   - Alcohol Wipes
   - Tissue Paper
   - Waste Bag
2. Check doctor's written order to perform laser PI in patient's medical notes.
3. Introduce self to patient.
4. Identify patient against medical record using at least 2 identifiers:
   - Patient Name
   - Patient Identification Number/Address/Date of Birth
5. Indicate the site for the procedure with the appropriate site marking sticker on patient's forehead.
   - For Right side—denoted by 'RIGHT' sticker.
   - For Left side—denoted by 'LEFT' sticker.
6. Familiarize yourself with laser settings and parameters.
7. Maintain patient comfort and positioning.
8. Monitor laser alignment and safety.
9. Document treatment details.
10. Prepare prescribed medication and perform a double check system, by 2 authorised personnel.
11. Check that the patient is not allergic to the drugs prescribed by verifying with the medical record and by asking the patient.
12. Ensure that the doctor explains to patient the purpose and any side effects and obtains consent from patient.

Performance Phase

1. Perform Time Out.
2. Perform hand wash/hand rub.
3. Prior to the Laser procedure, instil the following eye drops into patient's affected eye:
   - Gutt Pilocarpine 2% to constrict the pupil.

   - Gutt Brominidine to prevent post-laser IOP elevation if required.
   - Gutt Proparacaine 0.5% or Gutt/Minims Tetracaine 1% (topical anaesthetic drops) to anaesthetize the eye.
4. Wipe the essential parts of the machine that comes in contact with the patient with alcohol wipes before start of procedure.
5. Position patient comfortably in front of the Slit Lamp with chin and forehead resting firmly on the frame and strap patient's head before commencement of Laser procedure if necessary.
6. Doctor will perform the following:
   - Do site marking with skin marker during Time Out.
   - Place a Laser lens on the to direct the Laser light into the eye.
   - Perform the Laser treatment. Ensure patient's comfort after the Laser.
7. Wipe the essential parts of the machine that comes in contact with the patient with alcohol wipes after the procedure.
8. Perform hand wash/ hand rub.

Follow-Up Phase

1. Record the date and time of the Laser PI performed onto the patient's medical record.
2. Perform non-Contact tonometry to measure patient's eye pressure within 30 min to 1 h after Laser PI procedure to monitor any raise in IOP. Remove site marking sticker from patient's forehead.
3. Inform Doctor about patient's IOP (post laser) before discharging patient home.
4. Advise and issue information on post-laser procedure to patient.

5. Continue with the prescribed medication as advised by the doctor.
6. Advise patient on the follow-up review date.
7. Refer to Annexes Laser Treatment Checklist, and Post Laser Care and Advice.

> **GEH Perspectives**
> 1. Verify to correct patient, procedure, and site of procedure, ensuring informed consent has been obtained.
> 2. Ensure pupil is well dilated and maintain patient stability and positioning, using the appropriate laser protection goggles for assistants.
> 3. Monitor laser settings, alignment, and servicing of machine.
> 4. Ensure the patient understands possible side-effects, symptoms of complications and check post-procedure IOP.

Assisting in Retinal Argon Laser

Purpose

- To treat various Retinal Conditions such as Retinal Tears, Diabetic Retinopathy/Maculopathy, Proliferative Retinal Vascular Disorders, Central Serous Retinopathy, Choroidal Neovascularization and Chorioretinal Tumours.

Policy

- To establish standard procedure for Retinal Argon Laser.

Definition

1. Argon Laser is a Laser with ionized argon as the active medium, whose beam is in the blue and green visible light spectrum used for photocoagulation. Retinal photocoagulation procedures are one of the most common laser treatments performed and are usually done for advanced diabetic retinopathy.

Procedure

Preparatory Phase
1. Obtain appropriate requisites:
   - Mainster Lens—Standard/Widefield Lens
   - SuperQuad/Quadraspheric Lens
   - Vidisic Gel (Lens Lubricant)
   - Topical Anaesthetic Drops
     – Gutt/Minims Tetracaine 1%
     – Gutt Proparacine 0.5%
   - Dilating Eye Drops
     – Gutt Tropicamide 1%
     – Gutt Phenylephrine 2.5% (if required)
   - Laser Goggles
   - Alcohol Wipes
   - Tissue Paper
   - Waste Bag
2. Check doctor's written order to perform Retinal Argon Laser in patient's medical record.
3. Introduce self to patient.
4. Identify patient against medical record using at least 2 identifiers:
   - Patient Name
   - Patient Identification Number/Address/Date of Birth
5. Indicate the site for the procedure with the appropriate site marking sticker on patient's forehead.
   - For Right side—denoted by 'RIGHT' sticker.
   - For Left side—denoted by 'LEFT' sticker.

6. Prepare prescribed medication and perform a double check system, by 2 authorised personnel.
7. Observe the Guidelines on Administration of Medication (ref).
8. Check that the patient is not allergic to the drugs prescribed by verifying with the medical record and by asking the patient.
9. Ensure that the doctor explains to patient the purpose and any side effects and obtains consent from patient.

Performance Phase

1. Perform hand wash/hand rub.
2. Prior to the laser procedure, instil the following eye drops into patient's affected eye:
   - Gutt Tropicamide 1% to dilate the pupil.
   - Gutt Propracaine 0.5% or Gutt/Minims Tetracaine 1% (topical anaesthetic drops) to anaesthetize the eye.
3. Wipe the essential parts of the machine that comes in contact with the patient with alcohol wipes before start of procedure.
4. Position patient comfortably in front of the Slit Lamp with chin and forehead resting firmly on the frame and strap patient's head before commencement of Laser procedure if necessary.
5. Doctor will perform the following:
   - Do site marking with skin marker.
   - Place a Laser lens on the eye to direct the Laser light into the eye.
   - Perform the Laser treatment.
6. Ensure patient's comfort after the Laser.
7. Wipe the essential parts of the machine that comes in contact with the patient with alcohol wipes after the procedure.
8. Perform hand wash/ hand rub.

Follow-Up Phase

1. Record the date and time of the Argon Laser performed onto the patient's medical record.
2. Remove site marking sticker from patient's forehead.
3. Advise and issue information on post-laser procedure to patient.

4. Continue with the prescribed medication as advised by the doctor.
5. Advise patient on the follow-up review date.
6. Refer to Annexes Laser Treatment Checklist, and Post Laser Care and Advice.

> **GEH Perspectives**
> 1. Verify to correct patient, procedure, and site of procedure ensuring informed consent has been obtained.
> 2. Ensure pupil is well dilated and maintain patient stability and positioning using the appropriate laser protection goggles for assistants.
> 3. Monitor laser settings and alignment and proper servicing of machine.
> 4. Ensure the patient understands possible side-effects and symptoms of complications.

Annexes

Pre-laser Safety Checklist

DAILY LASER SAFETY CHECKLIST
(To be performed at the Start and End of the Day)

Month: _____

S/N	Checklist	Mon	Tue	Wed	Thu	Fri	Follow-Up Actions
AT THE START OF THE DAY							
1	Laser machine keys are retrieved from the designated locked storage and are accounted for.						
2	Laser machines / Slit Lamps are functioning well.						
(a)	Cables and bulbs are not damaged.						
(b)	Switches are working - Able to Turn ON / OFF.						
3	Laser Safety Goggles of appropriate wavelength and optical density are available in the laser room and are in good condition.						
4	Laser panel switch is ON and 'Laser In Progress' indicator light is functioning.						
5	'Request for Assistance' button in the laser room is functioning.						
6	Laser keys are removed from the machines and kept by the Laser Nurse in-Charge.						
7	Laser Lenses are checked - Inventory accounted for and lenses are cleaned, not scratched and damaged.						
8	Fire Extinguisher is readily available and within the validity period.						
	Checked By: (Name & Signature of Staff)						
S/N	Checklist	Mon	Tue	Wed	Thu	Fri	Follow-Up Actions

DAILY LASER SAFETY CHECKLIST						
(To be performed at the Start and End of the Day)						
						Month:
AT THE END OF THE DAY						
1	Laser machines / Slit Lamps are switched OFF and laser keys are removed from the machines.					
2	Laser machine keys are returned and kept in designated locked storage.					
3	Laser Lenses are cleaned, disinfected and stored in the cabinet dryer.					
4	Consumables, Stationaries, Clinical forms and Eyedrops / Ointments are replenished in all the laser rooms.					
5	Laser procedures done are recorded into the patient's Medical Record Notes and Laser Record Book.					
	Checked By: (Name & Signature of Staff)					

Note:
✓ Indicates item is checked and in order.
✗ Indicates item is NOT in order. To indicate on Follow-up Actions taken.

Table reproduced with permission and courtesy of SNEC.

Laser Treatment Checklist

LASER TREATMENT

Date : _____

Doctor : _____

Laser Room : _____

Patent Sticky Label

Site of Laser	RE	LE	BE

(Tick accordingly)

☐ NEW CASE Laser
☐ FOLLOW-UP REPEAT Laser (> 1 Year)
☐ LLOW-UP REPEAT Laser

	PRE-LASER CHECKLIST	YES	NO	NA	REMARKS
1	Check patient's identity				
2	Ensure Consent for Laser is taken and valid				
3	Check Validity of Laser Charges				
	☐ For NEW CASE Laser				
	⇨ Ensure that Laser Request form is duly completed				
	⇨				
	☐ For FOLLOW-UP REPEAT Laser (> 1 Year)				
	⇨ Ensure that Laser Request form is duly completed				
	☐ For FOLLOW-UP REPEAT Laser				
4	Indicate Eye for Laser ☐ RE ☐ LE ☐ BE				
5	Determine if Eye(s) need to be dilated				If Yes: ☐ RE ☐ LE ☐ BE
6	Set up DRG Form (For New & Follow-up Repeat Laser > 1 Yr)				

_____
(Name of Staff)

_____
(Signature)

	POST-LASER CHECKLIST	YES	NO	NA	REMARKS
1	Stamp 'Laser Done' onto patient's casenotes				
2	Stamp 'Laser Done' onto patient's Clinic Service Form (For Follow-up Repeat Laser only)				
3	Give Prescription Form to patient if required				
4	Give Post-Laser Information Advice				
5	Ensure DRG Form is duly completed by Doctor				
6	Send patient to the counter for Payment and Appointment				

_____
(Name of Staff)

_____
(Signature)

Table reproduced with permission and courtesy of SNEC.

Post-laser Care and Advice

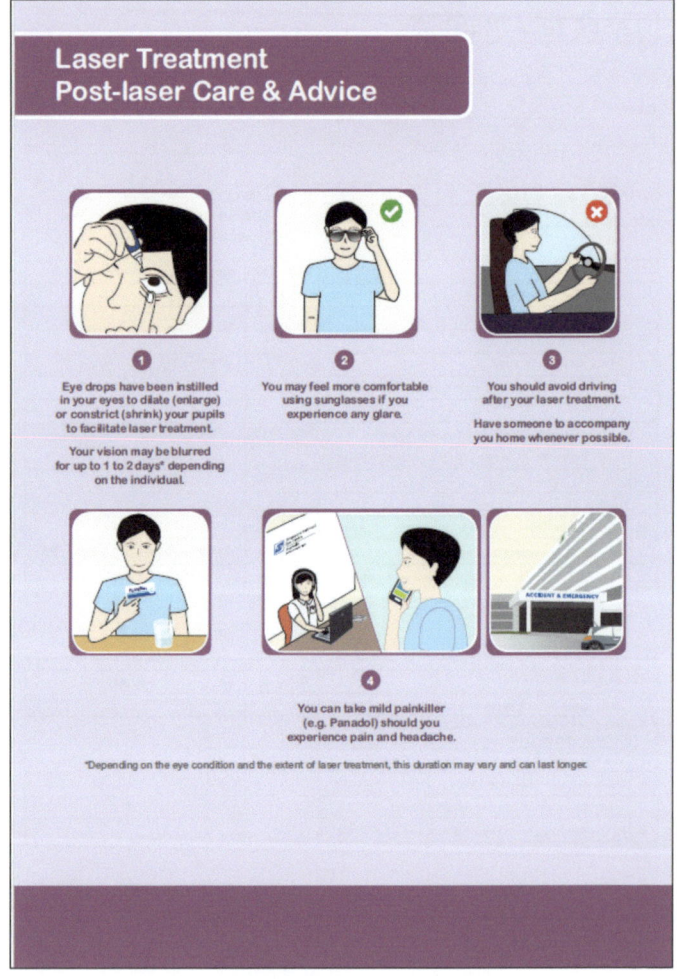

Images reproduced with permission and courtesy of SNEC.

Open Access This chapter is licensed under the terms of the Creative Commons Attribution-NonCommercial-NoDerivatives 4.0 International License (http://creativecommons.org/licenses/by-nc-nd/4.0/), which permits any noncommercial use, sharing, distribution and reproduction in any medium or format, as long as you give appropriate credit to the original author(s) and the source, provide a link to the Creative Commons license and indicate if you modified the licensed material. You do not have permission under this license to share adapted material derived from this chapter or parts of it.

The images or other third party material in this chapter are included in the chapter's Creative Commons license, unless indicated otherwise in a credit line to the material. If material is not included in the chapter's Creative Commons license and your intended use is not permitted by statutory regulation or exceeds the permitted use, you will need to obtain permission directly from the copyright holder.

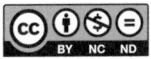

Endophthalmitis Prevention 54

Wiryasaputra Shaan and Chitra Vallei

Preoperative Measures

Optimize lid hygiene and ocular surface prior to listing for cataract surgery.

Instil 5% povidone-iodine to the cornea and conjunctival sac and clean peri ocular skin with 10% povidone-iodine. Ensure there is adequate contact time for microbicidal activity. Chlorhexidine 0.05% may be considered for patients with iodine allergies.

All instruments for surgery should be sterile. Consider disposable single use equipment where possible. Do not reuse items intended for single use.

Operating theatres should have in place separate clean and dirty circuits for all personnel and equipment. Quality assurance of air flow, temperature, humidity, ventilation, and surfaces should be performed periodically.

Endophthalmitis prevention and post-operative regime – adapted from ESCRS Guidelines for Prevention and Treatment of Endophthalmitis Following Cataract Surgery 2013.

W. Shaan · C. Vallei (✉)
Singapore National Eye Centre, Singapore Eye Research Institute, Singapore, Singapore
e-mail: wiryasaputra.shaan@singhealth.com.sg;
chitra.vallei@snec.com.sg

Drape the eye after cleaning, tape eyelids and lashes, prior to surgery.

Intraoperative Measures

Intracameral injection of antibiotics at the end of surgery in keeping with recommendations from the ESCRS Endophthalmitis Prophylaxis Study. The 2006/7 study demonstrated a 5-fold reduction in endophthalmitis rates in patients who received an intracameral injection of 1 mg cefuroxime at the close of surgery ($p = 0.001$ for presumed endophthalmitis; $p = 0.005$ for proven endophthalmitis).

Post-operative Measures

The post-operative treatment regime is influenced by multiple factors such as intra operative complications and pre-existing ocular surface disease. We favour the use of topical fluoroquinolones which have a broad spectrum of activity, good ocular penetration and minimal cornea toxicity.

> **GEH Perspectives**
> 1. Maintaining sterility is important while performing any surgical procedure.
> 2. Emphasis on hand hygiene for both staff and patients.
> 3. Patient education and emphasis on compliance of instillation of prescribed eye drops post procedure.

Reference

Endophthalmitis Study Group, European Society of Cataract & Refractive Surgeons, Prophylaxis of postoperative endophthalmitis following cataract surgery: results of the ESCRS multicenter study and identification of risk factors. J Cataract Refract Surg. 2007 33(6):978-88. doi: https://doi.org/10.1016/j.jcrs.2007.02.032

Open Access This chapter is licensed under the terms of the Creative Commons Attribution-NonCommercial-NoDerivatives 4.0 International License (http://creativecommons.org/licenses/by-nc-nd/4.0/), which permits any non-commercial use, sharing, distribution and reproduction in any medium or format, as long as you give appropriate credit to the original author(s) and the source, provide a link to the Creative Commons license and indicate if you modified the licensed material. You do not have permission under this license to share adapted material derived from this chapter or parts of it.

The images or other third party material in this chapter are included in the chapter's Creative Commons license, unless indicated otherwise in a credit line to the material. If material is not included in the chapter's Creative Commons license and your intended use is not permitted by statutory regulation or exceeds the permitted use, you will need to obtain permission directly from the copyright holder.

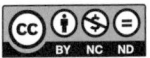

Refraction Protocol

55

Kothubutheen Mohamed Farook,
Lim Ling Yan, Li Fengxia,
and Lim Wei Lan Violet

Purpose

1. To document the visual function of the patient.
2. To determine the refractive error and/or other ocular anomalies.
3. To monitor the progression of the refractive error and the best corrected visual acuity (BCVA).

Definition

An assessment carried out by a trained certified professional on an individual to measure the refractive error and the best visual acuity.

Requisites

1. Room with adjustable illumination (preferred)
2. Visual Acuity Projector Chart or Digital Visual Acuity System
3. Retinoscope

K. M. Farook (✉) · L. L. Yan · L. Fengxia · L. W. L. Violet
Singapore National Eye Centre, Singapore Eye Research Institute,
Singapore, Singapore
e-mail: farook@snec.com.sg; lim.ling.yan@snec.com.sg;
li.fengxia@snec.com.sg; violet.lim.wl@snec.com.sg

© The Author(s) 2026
A. C S Tan et al. (eds.), *The Global Eye Health Handbook*,
https://doi.org/10.1007/978-981-96-8861-6_55

4. Trial Frames with a range of pupillary distance (PD)
5. Jackson Cross Cylinder (JCC) of various power
6. Near Reading Chart
7. PD Ruler
8. Focimeter/Lensmeter
9. Occluder with pinhole
10. Skiascopy lens rack
11. 70% isopropyl alcohol disinfectant wipes (To avoid use with any ophthalmic lenses)
12. Trial lens set

Instructions

Patient Preparation

1. Review the case history of patient.
2. Identify the correct patient using two patient identifiers.
3. Perform hand hygiene.
4. Explain the purpose of the test to the patient.
5. Ensure that the patient is seated comfortably on the examination chair at the calibrated distance from the projector/mirror.
    - Alternative use of Tumbling E and pictorial charts are to be considered for the patient who is unable to verbalise well.
    - Additional options to use Sheridan Gardiner or Kay picture chart for the paediatric patient unfamiliar with letters and/or numbers.
6. Discuss with the patient and/or the accompanying caregiver regarding the visual needs/requirements.
7. Assess the visual acuity (VA) (unaided/aided as pertinent) of the patient.
8. Document the details of optical aid such as spectacle type or contact lens used.

- Remove Bangerter foil or Fresnel prism if any, prior to the VA check.
- Present the VA chart in multiple linear lines whenever possible to simulate the crowding effect.

Procedures

1. Verify the prescription of the patient's spectacles, if any.
2. Measure the PD of patient (See Appendix A) and select a suitable trial frame size.

Retinoscopy

3. Select a suitable trial frame size as appropriate for the PD of the patient.
   - Add in appropriate fogging lens when performing retinoscopy.
4. Dim the room lighting if unable to obtain good visualisation of retinoscopy reflex.
5. Instruct patient to fixate at the target being shown at the VA chart.
   - Remind patient to alert the examiner if the target is being blocked.
6. Rotate the retinoscopy streak to align with the reflex power that is more positive/least minus.
7. Neutralise the meridian by adding PLUS lens for 'with movement' or MINUS lenses for 'against movement'.
8. Endpoint is obtained when there is a reversal in movement or when the reflex has reached a bright even glow (i.e. no motion).
9. Neutralise the next meridian by rotating the streak to 90° away from the first axis.
10. Repeat steps 7 and 8.
11. Final prescription of the patient is calculated by

- Removing the fogging lens from the trial lens or
- Removing the working distance power if skiascopy lens rack is used (e.g., remove +1.50DS for 67cm working distance)
12. Repeat steps 5–11 for the other eye.
13. Document any abnormalities of reflex noted (e.g. scissor reflex).

Types of retinoscopy reflexes

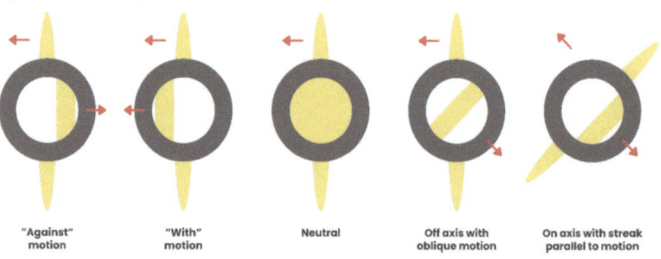

"Against" motion | "With" motion | Neutral | Off axis with oblique motion | On axis with streak parallel to motion

Figure Legend:

- *Against motion*: In myopic eye, "against light reflex" motion is seen. This would require a minus lens to neutralise the effect.
- *With motion*: In hyperopic eye, "with light reflex" motion is seen. This would require a plus lens to neutralise the effect.
- *Neutral* effect: Is seen when there is no obvious refractive error to be neutralised.
- *Off Axis with oblique motion*: Is seen when there is astigmatic correction to be neutralised but the retinoscopy reflex is not in alignment with the astigmatic axis to be neutralised.
- *On Axis with streak parallel to motion*: Indicates the astigmatic correction axis and the retinoscope light axis are in alignment.
- *Image reproduced with permission and courtesy of SNEC.*

Working distance calculation for retinoscopy:

Examiner/retinoscope distance	Working distance correction
50 cm	2.00 D
67 cm	1.50 D
100 cm	1.00 D

Subjective Refraction

14. Perform subjective refraction with appropriate room lighting by refining from the results of retinoscopy and/or autorefraction.

Determining Initial Best Vision Sphere

15. Occlude/fog the eye of the patient with the non-tested eye using an occluder or fogging lens. Fog with the appropriate plus lens for patients who are:
    - younger than 18 years of age
    - very accommodative
    - with nystagmus
16. Refine for initial best sphere from appropriate starting point considering retinoscopy/autorefraction readings and patient's condition.
    - Refine using ±0.25 spherical lenses.
    - Present the VA chart in multiple linear lines whenever possible to simulate the crowding effect.

Refining the Cylinder Axis and Power (Jackson Cross Cylinder)

17. Refine the retinoscopy astigmatism prescription using the Jackson Cross Cylinder (JCC).
    - Appropriate targets:
    - Clustered dots chart
    - Single line of letters or isolated optotype that is at least 2 sizes larger than the best sphere's visual acuity.
18. Minimum minus required for Maximum Visual Acuity (Final Best Vision Sphere). Refine the spherical power for BCVA using ±0.25 spherical lenses.
19. Repeat steps 14 and 18 to check the power of the other eye.
20. Perform binocular balancing (see Appendix B), where necessary.

Near Visual Acuity and Addition

21. Check monocular near vision and near addition power for patients:
    - ≥38 years old of age
    - With near visual complaints and/or
    - With conditions that can affect accommodation (e.g. pseudophakia, neuro-ophthalmological, atropine treatment, muscular disorder, etc.)
22. Ensure room illumination is sufficient and/or use a reading lamp.
23. Discuss the near visual targets and preferred/habitual reading distance with the patient.
24. Direct patient to hold the near VA chart at the preferred/habitual reading distance.
25. Measure the near visual acuity in each eye starting with a tentative addition power.

Age	Estimated ADD
40–45	+0.75 to +1.25
45–50	+1.25 to +1.75
50–55	+1.75 to +2.25
55–60	+2.25 to +2.50
>60	+2.50 or above

- Estimated near addition for post cataract surgery with monofocal intraocular lens implant is approximately +2.50DS at the distance of 40 cm.
26. Refine the near addition power by requesting the patient to compare with ±0.25 D spherical lens.
27. Determine the range of clear vision with the near addition power.
    - Instruct patient to bring the reading chart towards and away from him/her until the target becomes blurry to determine the range.
    - Check the range of clear vision again binocularly.
28. Record the result of refraction with near addition power and VA.

Follow-Up Phase

1. Formulate a management plan and discuss with the patient regarding the feasibility of plan, prescription of optical aids (if necessary) and/or clarify any concerns. Document what was transpired to the patient.

Appendix

Distance PD Measurement

Binocular PD Measurement
1. Ensure that the patient's head is positioned upright.
2. Examiner to be positioned at eye-level in front of the patient.
3. Rest the PD ruler gently on the patient's nose.
4. Instruct patient to look at examiner's left open eye (right eye closed).
5. Align the zero marking with the temporal limbus of the patient's right eye.
6. Instruct patient to look at examiner's right open eye (left eye closed).
7. Record the readings on the PD ruler's scale aligned with the nasal limbus of the patient's left eye.

Binocular Balance

Binocular Balancing Alternate Occlusion Technique (Patient with Equal BCVA)
1. Add +0.75DS on both eyes and present the 6/9 line for patients with BCVA of 6/6 in both eyes.
2. Alternate cover each eye while asking the patient to determine if either one eye is clearer than the other.

3. Add +0.25DS to the clearer eye to fog it further.
4. Repeat and compare the clarity of each eye again.
5. Stop when the clarity of each eye appears to be the same or when there is a reversal.
6. Recheck the subjective refraction if the clearer eye remains clear even after adding >+0.75DS.

Humphriss Immediate Contrast Technique (Patient with Equal or Unequal BCVA)

1. Fog the left eye with +1.00 DS.
2. Perform BVS in the right eye by asking the patient to read the best VA line.
3. Add +0.25 DS and ask patient if the letters are clearer, blurrier or the same.
4. Add +0.25 DS if the VA is the same or better.
5. Continue to add +0.25 DS until the VA worsens. (The sphere power is the prescription before the drop in VA)
6. Remove the +1.00 DS lens and now place it in front of the right eye.
7. Repeat steps 2–5 for the left eye with right eye fogged with +1.00DS.

> **GEH Perspectives**
> 1. During refraction, it is useful to understand the holistic nature of what might be relevant to affect a refraction outcome. This could include previous and existing eye and health conditions, to previous and existing visual aids, to visual requirements and lifestyle. (I.e. visual requirements of taxi driver, lorry driver, lecturer requiring distance, intermediate and near vision simultaneously)

2. It is helpful to identify end points to achieve the best vision sphere and cylinder power between and within optometrists to ensure consistency.
3. It is useful to access suitability of different types of optical aids (including its pros and cons), likelihood of adaptation and level of benefit for patients across different age groups. This is done in consideration of the individual's budget and what is available in the market.

References

Cynthia Matossian. (2017). Lessons learned in adapting EDOF IOLs. Available: https://www.ophthalmologytimes.com/view/lessonslearned-adapting-edof-iols. Last accessed 21st March 2021.

Hamed Momeni-Moghaddam and David A Goss. (2014). Comparison of four different binocular balancing techniques. Clinical and Experimental Optometry. 97 (5), 422-425.

Louise Wood. (2020). Intraocular Lenses: Navigating the Options. Available: https://www.mieducation.com/pages/intraocularlenses-navigating-the-options. Last accessed 28th Mar 2021.

Mark E Wilkinson. (2016a). General Refraction Techniques. Available: https://webeye.ophth.uiowa.edu/eyeforum/video/Refraction/pdfs/Stdsubj-Refract-Plus-Cyl-Tech-s.pdf. Last accessed 28th Mar 2021.

Mark E Wilkinson. (2016b). Sharpen your Subjective Refraction Technique. Available: https://www.reviewofoptometry.com/article/sharpen-your-subjectiverefraction-technique. Last accessed 21 Mar 2021.

Richard J. Kolker. (2014). Subjective Refraction and Prescribing Glasses. Available: http://www.aao.org/Assets/563fc40b-1466-477ebc12-4e62f8b2d324/635476894936870000/subjective-refractionprescribing-glasses-pdf. Last accessed 18th Mar 2021

Open Access This chapter is licensed under the terms of the Creative Commons Attribution-NonCommercial-NoDerivatives 4.0 International License (http://creativecommons.org/licenses/by-nc-nd/4.0/), which permits any non-commercial use, sharing, distribution and reproduction in any medium or format, as long as you give appropriate credit to the original author(s) and the source, provide a link to the Creative Commons license and indicate if you modified the licensed material. You do not have permission under this license to share adapted material derived from this chapter or parts of it.

The images or other third party material in this chapter are included in the chapter's Creative Commons license, unless indicated otherwise in a credit line to the material. If material is not included in the chapter's Creative Commons license and your intended use is not permitted by statutory regulation or exceeds the permitted use, you will need to obtain permission directly from the copyright holder.

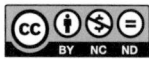

For Imaging Specialists

Patrick Ng Yuen Hwa
and Hlaing Thandar Aung

Minimum Standards for Biometry for Choosing Intraocular Lens

Biometry Techniques

- Use optical biometry to measure the axial length of the eye for people having cataract surgery
- Use ultrasound biometry if optical biometry
    - Is not possible **or**
    - Does not give accurate measurements
- Use keratometry to measure the curvature of the cornea for people having cataract surgery.
- Consider corneal topography for people having cataract surgery:
    - Who have abnormally flat or steep corneas
    - Who have irregular corneas
    - Who have significant astigmatism
    - Who have had previous corneal refractive surgery **or**
    - If it is not possible to get an accurate keratometry measurement

Biometry Formulas

- For people who have not had previous corneal refractive surgery, use 1 of the following to calculate the intraocular lens power before cataract surgery:
  - If the axial length is less than 22.00 mm, use Haigis or Hoffer Q.
  - If the axial length is between 22.00 and 26.00 mm, use Barrett Universal II if it is installed on the biometry device and does not need the results to be transcribed by hand. Use SRK/T if not.
  - If the axial length is more than 26.00 mm, use Haigis or SRK/T.
- Advise people who have had previous corneal refractive surgery that refractive outcomes after cataract surgery are difficult to predict, and that they may need further surgery if they do not want to wear spectacles for distance vision.
- If people have had previous corneal refractive surgery, adjust for the altered relationship between the anterior and posterior corneal curvature. Do not use standard biometry techniques or historical data alone.
- Surgeons should think about modifying a manufacturer's recommended intraocular lens constant, guided by learning gained from their previous deviations from predicted refractive outcomes.

Second-Eye Prediction

Consider using 50% of the first-eye prediction error in observed refractive outcome to guide calculations for the intraocular lens power for second-eye cataract surgery.

NICE guidelines do not stipulate when biometry should be repeated, 2010 FRCOPhth College guidelines recommends repeating biometry when:

- Axial length under 21.2 mm or over 26.6 mm
- Mean keratometry under 41D or over 47D
- Corneal astigmatism over 2.5D
- Difference in axial length between fellow eyes over 0.7 mm
- Difference in mean keratometry between fellow eyes over 0.9D

Standard Biometry Practices and Workflows

Biometry, A-Scan and B-Scan

Patients referred for A-scan ultrasound biometry and B-scan investigations will have accurate measurements taken and recorded.

Biometry of the eye refers to the measurement of various dimensions of the eye and of its components and their interrelationship. This includes axial length (AL) measurement, keratometry readings (corneal power), anterior chamber depth, lens thickness, white to white measurement and selection of IOL formulae to ensure accurate biometry. AXL AL error of 1 mm can cause a post-operative refractive error of approximately of 2.5–2.0D.

Introduction

The A scan, also defined as amplitude scan, measure the distance between structures of the eye (cornea to retina surface). It uses single beam, linear waves to produce a one-dimensional display spike.

It is commonly known as axial length and should be used together with other biometric measurement of the eye and IOL formulae to calculate IOL power for cataract surgery.

A scan can also be used for diagnosis e.g., the characteristics of mass in the eye reflected with the intensity of the spike.

Methods Used
- Applanation biometry (different brands available in the market)
- Immersion biometry (different brands available in the market)

Resources
- Applanation or Immersion Biometry machine such as vupad AB Scan, Vumax AB Scan, Ocuscan RxP, etc.
- A Scan and B Scan probe
- Alcohol wipes to wipe down B Scan Probe
- Anioxyde (3% hydrogen peroxide) solution to disinfect the A Scan probe and Prager shell.
- Sterile water (2 separate cups): one for rinsing after scan and another for after disinfection with Anioxyde. The first cup can be identified with a sticker.
- BSS bottle, Prager shell, tubing kit for water immersion
- Reclinable chair (optional) for water immersion
- Proparacaine 0.5% eye drop
- External printer
- Ultrasound transmission gel for B Scan

Process

Preparation
Ensure safety by checking that machine wires and cables are tucked safely away from patient.

Prepare Equipment for Keratometry Readings
- Switch on Keratometer and set to K reading mode.
- Select either manual or automatic mode of keratometry (e.g. Topcon Auto-refracto-keratometer KR8900).
- Clean chin and head rests with alcohol wipe.

Prepare for A Scan and B Scan
- Switch on machine.
- Ensure A scan and B scan probes are connected to the machine.
- Ensure that food pedal is plugged to the machine.

- Do a functionality and probe sensitivity check on A Scan machine using the built-in eye model cylinder block. Inform vendor if the reading is out of the range (usually 10.00 mm ± 0.10 mm).
- Introduce self to patient and verify patient's identity to ensure correct patient.
- Confirm Biometry request form for instruction or any special test or lens ordered by doctor.
- Explain the purpose and procedure to patients to allay fear and anxiety.
- Ensure patient's comfort and seek patient's co-operation.

Administrating the Test

Enter Patient's Data into the Machine

Perform Keratometer Reading (K-reading)
- Position patient comfortably on the chair facing keratometer.
- Adjust table height according to patient's sitting height so that patient will be able to rest their chin and forehead comfortably without straining forward. Body movement will be minimized.
- Position patient's chin on the chin rest and forehead against the headrest.
- Alight patient's eye level appropriately.
- Advise patient to focus on the centre of the picture.
- Align machine to the correct eye.
- Press trigger on joystick to capture K reading measurements.
- Print results after taking 3 consistent K readings.
- Interpret reliability of K reading results.
- Enter the K reading results into ultrasound machine.

Perform Contact Applanation A-Scan
- Position patient comfortably on the chair in front of the machine.
- Verify with patient if there is any drug allergy.
- Instil Proparacaine 0.5% into both eyes.
- Adjust gain control and ensure correct mode is used.

- Inform patient that the A scan probe will be touching his cornea during the procedure.
- Inform patient on appropriate fixation.
- Step on the foot pedal to start the measurement taking.
- Several measurements are to be taken.
- Evaluate and observe echo pattern during the procedure.
- Allow patient to blink eyes in between measurements.
- Print out A scan spike and IOL calculations based on surgeon's A constant.
- Wash the used probe in sterile water first cup and soak the A scan probe in Anioxyde solution for 5 min. Then rinse off in another cup of sterile water and dry the probe with optical lens fibre wipes or clean tissues and keep it in the probe holder (Fig. 56.1).

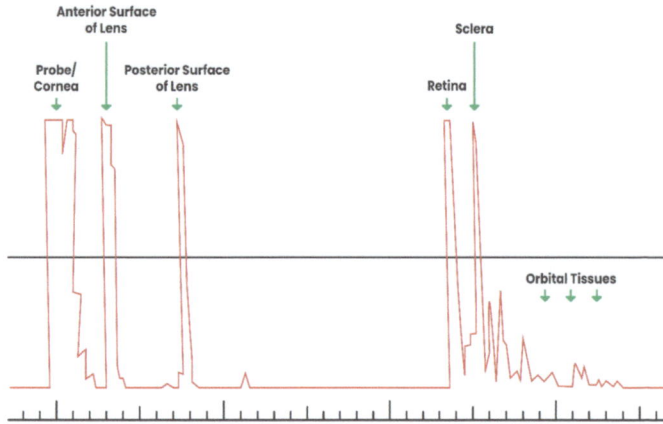

Fig. 56.1 High quality contact applanation ultrasound A-scan spike of phakic eye. Note 5 high-amplitude spikes and perpendicular retinal spike. Also, good resolution of separate retinal and scleral spikes is seen followed by orbital tissues. To obtain a minimum of 5 consistent Axial length measurements with maximum Standard Deviation of 0.05. *Image reproduced courtesy of SNEC.*

Perform Water Immersion A-Scan

- Position patient comfortably on the reclinable chair.
- Explain to patient the procedure will be conducted when patient is examined in a supine position looking at the ceiling.
- Verify with patient if there is any drug allergy.
- Instil Proparacaine 0.5% into both eyes.
- Adjust gain control and ensure immersion mode is used.
- Insert immersion A scan probe into Prager shell and tighten the gap between them.
- Connect tubing kit and BSS bottle to Prager shell.
- Inform patient to fixate both eyes at the ceiling.
- Inform patient that a Prager shell will be inserted and place under the eyelids and then filled with BSS solution.
- Step on the foot pedal to start the measurement taking. Several measurements are to be taken.
- Evaluate and observe echo pattern during the procedure.
- Observe the measurements taken.
- Remove the Prager shell and adjust patient to a sitting position.
- Print out A scan spike and IOL calculations based on the surgeon's A- constant.
- Wash the used probe and Prager shell in sterile water first cup and soak them in Anioxyde solution for 5 min. Then rinse off in another cup of sterile water and dry them with optical lens fibre wipes or clean tissues and keep the probe in the probe holder and the Prager shell on the clean rubber (to prevent damage) in the clean stainless stain container (to prevent cross infection) (Fig. 56.2).

Perform B-Scan

- Position patient comfortably on the chair in front of the machine.
- Advise patient to look straight in front.
- Adjust gain control.
- Inform patient of the B-Scan probe being placed on the eye during procedure.
- Apply ultrasound transmission gel on the tip of B scan Probe.

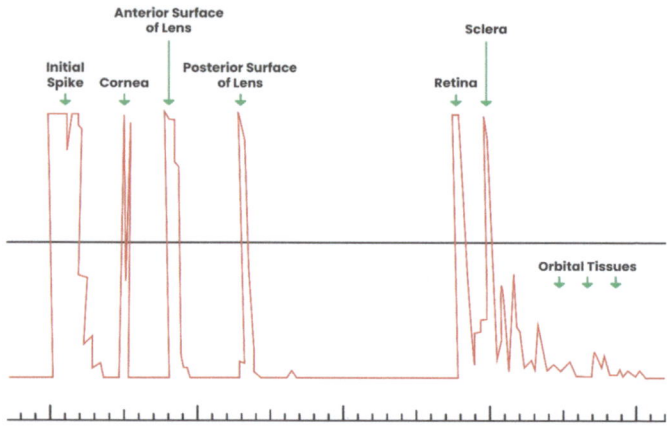

Fig. 56.2 High quality water immersion ultrasound A-scan spike of phakic eye. The probe and the cornea are now separate spikes because they are not in contact with each other. To obtain a minimum of 5 consistent Axial length measurements with maximum Standard Deviation of 0.05. *Image reproduced courtesy of SNEC.*

- Scan, observe the dynamic movement of the eye and freeze the appropriate image with the foot pedal with labelling of the scan image.
- Select and print the appropriate image with labelling.
- Repeat the scan if required.
- Clean gel from patient's eye with clean tissue after scanning.
- Wipe down and disinfect the probe with alcohol wipes. For infectious cases, use Virusolve+ to disinfect the probe.

File results into patient's medical record folder. To ensure good quality of biometry performed, the setup of an internal workflow should be implemented.

Switch off machine at the end of each session.

Place dust cover over machine at the end of the clinic.

Maintenance

Disconnect equipment from its power source before the start of servicing to avoid electrical shock.

Inspect cables, switches, and connections to ensure that they are not damaged.

Clean the main body of the equipment and the foot pedal with a dry and soft cloth to ensure that no moisture will penetrate the equipment.

Clean the equipment housing with a dry and soft cloth. Perform disinfection of the probes with the followings.

(a) A- Scan probe—with Anioxyde and rinse with sterile water. Dry the tip with clean tissue or optical lens fiber wipes and keep it in the probe holder.
(b) B- Scan probe—with alcohol wipes or virusolve+ wipes.

Connect equipment to its power source and test that equipment is functioning.

Perform Calibration of the equipment:

(a) Follow the manufacturer system calibration protocol to calibrate the probe. Usually, the A scan machine comes with built in eye model calibration cylinder block for system calibration.
(b) Adjust and hold the probe as perpendicular as possible to the top surface, to generate and receive an echo of maximum strength from the bottom surface.
(c) Ensure that cylinder calibration reading is within 10 mm (±) 0.1 mm (subject to manufacturer recommendation/handbook or manual).
(d) Dry the probe tip and test block surface with cotton swab and place probe in holder.
(e) If calibration cannot be verified, contact vendor to report on the abnormality.

Place dust cover over the equipment after servicing.

Optical Biometry

Patients referred for optical biometry investigations will have accurate measurements of Axial length, cornea curvature, Anterior chamber depth and white-to-white taken and recorded.

Introduction
A combined biometry instrument that measures parameters of the human eye needed for intraocular lens calculation.

Use optical partial coherence interferometry for measurement.

Emits an infrared laser beam that is reflected back to the instrument from the retinal pigment epithelium.

The reflected light is received by the instrument and axial length is calculated using a modified Michelson interferometer.

Resources
- Optical biometer such as IOL master 500 machine, IOL 700 machine, Topcon Aladdin, etc.
- Alcohol wipes
- External printer
- Barcode scanner (optional) to scan patient IC to prevent from human error or efficiency

Process

Preparation
Switch on the machine. The IOL master 500 will start performing self-test.

Ensure safety by checking that machine wires and cables are tucked safely away from patient.

Clean surface of machine with alcohol wipes to minimize risk of cross infection.

Introduce self to patient and verify patient's identity to ensure correctness.

Confirm doctor's request on the test required.

Explain the purpose and procedure to patient to allay fear and anxiety.

Ensure patient's comfort and seek patient's co-operation.

Dim the room light before procedure.

Administrating the test (For IOL master 500)

Enter patient's data and other required information into the machine.

Position patient comfortably on the chair facing the acquisition unit.

Adjust the table height according to patient's sitting height so that patient will be able to rest their chin and forehead comfortably without straining forward. Body movement will be minimized.

Advise patient to place chin on the chin rest and forehead against the forehead strap.

Adjust chin rest until patient's eye level is aligned with the two red ring marks on the side of the headrest.

Perform Procedure on Right Eye First

- Align the instrument to the patient's eye using the joystick via overview mode.
- Ask patient to focus on the centre fixation light. In ALM mode, the fixation light is red, otherwise it is always yellow.

Axial Length Measurement (ALM)

- Activate ALM mode using the mouse or pushbutton on the joystick.
- Default mode will be in phakic setting. To change setting, select the corresponding mode from the AL setting Eye status' menu.
- Ask patient to look at the red fixation light.
- A crosshair with a circle in the middle appears on the display.
- Further align the instrument so that the reflection of the alignment light appears within the circle.
- Start the measurement using the pushbutton on the joystick.
- Each eye measurement can display up to 20 readings, but the measurement is unlimited.

Measurement of Corneal Curvature
- Activate by pressing the <space> bar or the appropriate button.
- Ask patient to look at the yellow light.
- Move the centre point to the centre of the crosshair and align the device such that all 6 peripheral measurement points are arranged symmetrically around the crosshair, are within the circle and are as sharp as possible.
- Advise patient to blink eye shortly before the measurement to procedure adequate tear film, this will improve the reflectivity of the cornea.
- Start the measurement by pressing the button on the joystick.
- If a measurement point is not correctly detected, a blue flashing point will be indicated. Continue to perform a new measurement.
- 3 measurements are automatically taken. Measurements may be repeated if the readings are inconsistent or standard deviation is too large.

Anterior Chamber Depth Measurement (ACD)
- Activate the ACD mode via the <space> bar.
- The system will automatically turn on lateral slit illumination.
- Ask patient to look at the yellow fixation light.
- Carry out fine adjustment so that the fixation point is visible within the rectangle on the display and in the sharpest possible focus.
- The fixation point must be situated between the optical sections of the cornea and crystalline lens, as close as possible to (but not touching) the optical section of the crystalline lens (the cornea will appear out of focus).
- Start the measurement using the push button on the joystick.
- Values are recorded and displayed per measurement. The mean value is used for the IOL calculation.
- The ACD measurements may be repeated if necessary.

White-to-White (WTW) Measurement
- Activate the WTW mode via the <space> bar.
- Ask patient to look at the yellow fixation light.

- Adjust the device so that the 6 illumination LEDS are centred symmetrically around the crosshair and the iris structure/edge of pupil are in focus.
- Start the measurement suing the pushbutton on the joystick.
- WTW measurements may be repeated if necessary.

Confirm the obtained results and print the measurement results.
Repeat procedures for the left eye.
IOL calculation

- Use the IOL master to generate IOL options base on all the measured values.
- Click on the appropriate tab to select the desired formula.
- Select the appropriate lens from available lens types.
- Print out the calculated data by clicking the "print IOL calculation data" button.

File data into patient's medical folder.
Perform data back-up from hard disk to external or shared folder on a weekly basis if possible.
Disinfect machine with alcohol wipes after each patient's use.
Switch off the machine at the end of each session.
Place dust cover over machine at the end of each session.

Maintenance

Disconnect/switch off equipment from its power source before the start of servicing to avoid electrical shock.

Inspect cables, bulbs, switches, and connections to ensure that they are not damaged.

Clean the equipment housing with a dry and soft cloth to ensure that no moisture will penetrate the equipment. The equipment housing includes:

(a) Adjustable table
(b) Motorized stand
(c) Joystick
(d) Chin rest/handle

(e) Forehead rest
(f) Barcode scanner

Disinfect the chin rest/Handle and forehead rest with alcohol wipes.

Connect equipment to its power source and test that equipment is functioning.

Perform measurement verification of the equipment:

(a) User the "test eye" model to verify the accuracy of measurement.
(b) Place the test eye model on the holding pins beside the chin rest and perpendicular in front of the equipment.
(c) Select patient list as "measure function check" and click "new".
(d) Select "Test Eye" from the options menu and the word "Test Eye" will be displayed.
(e) Measure the "Test Eye" labelled with AL and R for testing Axial length mode and keratometer (R). The tolerance range must be within the range indicated on the eye model itself.
(f) Measure the "Test Eye" labelled with ACD/VKT for testing the anterior chamber depth mode. The tolerance range must be within the range indicated on the eye model itself.
(g) Print the results for record.
(h) If the measurement cannot be verified, contact vendor to report on the abnormality.

Place dust cover over the equipment after servicing.

Biometry Parameters

Parameters	Axial Length (AXL)	Axial Length (AXL) Remark	K-reading	K-reading Remark	Anterior Chamber Depth (ACD)	White-to-White (WTW)	IOL Formula
Equipments							
1. Optical biometry							
1.1 IOL Master v5.4	min 6, average 10 reading	Quality of tower by referring to operating manual	min 3 reading	Repeatability between two equipment by comparing with Auto-K. K-reading difference by ±0.25 is acceptable.	Repeatability of reading	Repeatability of reading	Provide SRKT formula Additional HofferQ Formula for AXL ≤22 mm Additional Haigis Formula for AXL ≥26 mm
1.2 IOL Master 500 v 7.5	SNR ≥1.6				Repeatability of reading	Repeatability of reading	
1.3 IOL Master 700	min 6 reading SD ≥27 μm	Based on manufacturer guidelines by using the traffic light during measurement.					Provide Barette formula

(continued)

Parameters	Axial Length (AXL)	Axial Length (AXL) Remark	K-reading	K-reading Remark	Anterior Chamber Depth (ACD)	White-to-White (WTW)	IOL Formula
2. *Ultrasound Biometry*							
	min 5 reading	(a) To review on the quality of the A-scan spikes.	3 consistent readings with average K1 & K2 readings input into the Ultrasound Equipment	Repeatability between two equipment by comparing with Auto-K. K-reading difference by ±0.25 is acceptable	Repeatability of reading		Provide SRKT formula
	SD ≤0.05 mm	(b) Compare with other equipment based on the clinic settings					Additional HofferQ Formula for AXL ≤22 mm
							Note. Do not provide Haigis Forumla for AXL ≥26 mm as Haigis Formula is not optimized for Ultrasound method

Table reproduced with permission and courtesy of SNEC
NOTE 1. If unable to obtain measurement from any optical methods, to opt for Ultrasound method
NOTE 2. In the event where encountered any doubts, please indicate comments and refer to surgeon

General Remarks

1. All equipment should be verified using manufacturer eye model on daily basis.
2. All equipment Preventive Maintenance should be carried out by vendor based on their recommended frequency.
3. All probes that is in contact with patients should be disinfected by approved disinfectant, Anioxyde1000.
4. All Optical Biometer's ULIB A-constant should be updated half yearly.
5. All Biometry Report are valid for 6months from the date of performing.
6. Always perform K-reading first before any contact of the eye. And Lubricant for post operation.
7. Always perform optical biometry as the 1st method.
8. Lubricate the eyes with poor mires when performing biometry and keratometry
9. Pay attention to details such as chin and head rest.
10. Repeat the test if necessary to minimize refractive surprises.

Axial Length (AXL)

1. Always measure Both Eye AXL for phakic eye and document it in report.
2. In the event where the difference is >0.5 mm, to compare with other equipment. Or perform B Scan to check if any abnormalities.

K-reading

1. For contact lens wearer, to off soft contact lens for 7 days & hard contact lens for 14 days.
2. For any cornea diseases (PK, cornea transplant, cornea scar), unable to obtain K-reading measurement:

- Use K1 = 44D, K2 = 44D
- Use K reading of the other phakic eye.
- Any difficulties obtaining K-reading, please refer to the surgeon.

Post-refractive Surgery Cases

1. OU Biometry should be performed.
2. Cornea mapping should also be performed for both eyes.
3. Haigis-L/Haigis-Suite Formula should be given with the correct refractive status of the eye. Barette Formula to be given for IOL 700 biometer.

IOL Formula

1. For any complicated cases, please refer to surgeon.
2. For normal cases, please refer to the table in 3.3.

Three Roles of Biometry

Each role is required to ensure accuracy and consistency of IOL selection:

- Performer
- Checker 1
- Checker 2

Role of Biometry Performer

1. Ensure that *Patients' Particulars* (Name, Identity number, D.O.B, address) are correct.
2. Verify *Operating Eye and Ocular history verification*. (Contact lens, refractive surgery)

3. Perform *biometry* according to completed biometry request form (Auto keratometry, Axial length, ACD, WTW). Ensure consistency and accuracy, repeat or double check the measurements whenever in doubt.
   - To refer to surgeon for clarification/verification when necessary.
4. Highlight any *abnormalities* affecting biometric measurement that require attention and flag to surgeon for attention.
5. Perform *IOL Calculation* printout & lens reservation.

Role of Biometry Checker 1

1. Ensure that *Patients' Particulars* (Name, Identity number, D.O.B, address) are correct.
2. Ensure that any *abnormalities* affecting biometric measurement that require attention are flagged by performer to surgeon for attention.
3. Ensure that biometry is performed accordingly to biometry checklist and biometry equipment parameter.
4. Ensure that IOL calculation printout includes the selection of *IOL to be implanted* (if any specific premium lens is requested) in the biometry request form.
5. Check and sign according to *Biometry Checklist* after biometry is performed.

Role of Biometry Checker 2

1. Ensure that *Patients' Particulars* (Name, Identity number, D.O.B, address) are correct.
2. Ensure that any *abnormalities* affecting biometric measurement that require attention are flagged by performer to surgeon for attention.
3. Ensure that biometry is performed accordingly to biometry checklist and biometry equipment parameter.

4. Ensure that IOL calculation printout includes the selection of *IOL to be implanted* (if any specific premium lens is requested) in the biometry request form.
5. Check and sign according to *Biometry Checklist* after biometry is performed.
6. Review consistency of IOL implant of operated eye (*If applicable*).

> **GEH Perspectives for Optimal Biometry Results**
> 1. Always perform keratometry and optical biometry before instillation of eyedrops or stains and before procedure that requires direct eye contact.
> 2. Repeat the test when in doubt or compare and double check with other modality to ensure consistency and accuracy of the measurement. Always good to compare biometry of the fellow eye for reference and consistency.
> 3. Calibration and preventive maintenance of biometry and keratometry equipment should be performed according to manufacturer or vendor guideline to ensure accuracy and functionality of equipment.
> 4. Hand-hygiene and disinfection of equipment and related accessories (e.g. probes) must be performed according to infection control protocol.
> 5. It is good to implement checker protocol to check the performer work after biometry to minimise discrepancy and inaccuracy in biometry and IOL calculation due to human errors.

References

Demonstration on IOL 500 usage. https://youtu.be/Hvq51Ttbj6w?si=EOXIsFA5g8hm5hVd

Demonstration on IOL 700 usage. (72) ZEISS IOLMaster 700 – Tutorial – Measurement and Analysis – YouTube https://www.youtube.com/watch?v=0KzGDNfYZWs

Ashok Garg, J.T. Lin, Robert Latkany, Jerome Bovet, Wolfgang Haigis (2009). Mastering the techniques of IOL power calculations, 2nd edition.

Sonomed Escalon. Operator's manual- EZ scan AB5500. Lake success, USA: Sonomed Escalon; ND.

Carl Zeiss Meditec AG. Operators' manual- IOL master 2015. Available from: http://www.doctor-hill.com/iol-master/iolmaster_tutorial.html.

Millodot M. Dictionary of optometry and visual science. 7th edition. London: Butterworth Heinemann Elsevier; 2008

Alcon Laboratories I. OcuScan ® RxP Measuring system. Operator's manual. Forth worth, USA: Alcon Laboratories, INC.; ND.

Mandarin Opto-Medic Co Pte Ltd. Operator's manual – A2500 A-scan. Singapore: Mandarin opto-medic Co Pte Ltd; ND.

Patrick Ng, Eileen Lim, Aw Ai Tee, Eunice Loh, Margaret Tan, Vicky Drury (2007). Procedure manual of ophthalmic investigations. https://emedicine.medscape.com/article/1228447-overview?form=fpf#a2

Diagnostic testing: A-scan biometry. The Eye Institute for Medicine & Surgery. Available at https://www.seebetterbrevard.com/diagnostic-testing/ascan.php. Accessed: June 6, 2022.

Open Access This chapter is licensed under the terms of the Creative Commons Attribution-NonCommercial-NoDerivatives 4.0 International License (http://creativecommons.org/licenses/by-nc-nd/4.0/), which permits any non-commercial use, sharing, distribution and reproduction in any medium or format, as long as you give appropriate credit to the original author(s) and the source, provide a link to the Creative Commons license and indicate if you modified the licensed material. You do not have permission under this license to share adapted material derived from this chapter or parts of it.

The images or other third party material in this chapter are included in the chapter's Creative Commons license, unless indicated otherwise in a credit line to the material. If material is not included in the chapter's Creative Commons license and your intended use is not permitted by statutory regulation or exceeds the permitted use, you will need to obtain permission directly from the copyright holder.

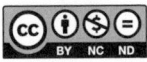

Focus on Cataract Outcomes

Ralene Sim

Reference: Report of the 2030 targets on effective coverage of eye care (World Health Organization, 2022. ISBN978-92-4-005800-2)

World Health Organisation (WHO) definition of standards for the outcomes of cataract surgery—three categories:

1. Good (postoperative visual acuity outcome better than 6/12)
2. Borderline (visual acuity outcome in the range 6/12–6/60)
3. Poor (visual acuity less than 6/60)

WHO recommendations for acceptable outcomes at 1-day post-operation are:

4. 40% cases achieving acuity between 6/6 and 6/18 (Good result).
5. 50% of cases achieving a visual acuity between 6/24 and 6/60 (Borderline result).
6. No more than 10% cases at less than 6/60 (poor result) with half of those due to intraoperative complications.
7. In many situations it is difficult to obtain follow-up at 6–8 weeks, but by then the recommendations have risen to

R. Sim (✉)
Department of Training and Education, Singapore National Eye Centre, Singapore Eye Research Institute, Singapore, Singapore
e-mail: ralene.sim@mohh.com.sg

85% of cases with a good outcome and only 5% with a poor outcome.

Factors determining surgical outcome include ocular co-morbidity, the availability of preoperative biometry, surgical expertise/facilities, and correction of residual refractive error.

Phaco Outcomes from Studies

- National data on the results of phacoemulsification surgery in the UK and Western Europe: >80% of patients achieve a final VA of 6/12 or better with a complication rate of 4%.
- Eastern Africa and India: wide variation in final visual acuity ranging between 38 and 80% of patients achieving 6/18 or better with a complication rate between 7 and 20% of cases.

(However, many of these studies include patients undergoing extracapsular, intracapsular and even couching procedures, so direct comparisons are not possible)

SICS Outcomes from Studies

- *Rupak KJ et al., 2023*: 315 patients from South Gujarat, India
  Participants were categorized according to the WHO criteria into four groups having visual acuity <3/60, 3/60–5/60, 6/60–6/18, and >6/18. Out of 315, 205 (*65.08%*) patients had preoperative vision <3/60, whereas only 5 (1.59%) had vision >6/18. Postoperatively, 302 (95.87%) achieved vision better than 6/18.
- *Jay JM et al., 2020*: Compare visual outcomes of SICS and phacoemulsification.
  705 eyes studied (509 phaco, 196 SICS) from New Zealand.
  At the early post-operative visit, a higher proportion in the phaco group achieved $\geq$6/18 UCVA (81.5% phaco vs *64.8%* SICS, $p < 0.0001$) and BCVA (87.8% phaco vs. 73.5% SICS, $p < 0.0001$).

At the late post-operative visit, a higher proportion following phaco also achieved ≥6/18 UCVA (93.9% phaco vs. *85.2%* SICS, $p = 0.0004$) and BCVA (96.9% phaco vs. *91.3%* SICS, $p = 0.004$). After exclusion of eyes with pre-existing ocular comorbidities, a similar proportion had ≥6/18 late UCVA (98.9% phaco vs. 96.9% SICS, $p = 0.22$) and BCVA (100% phaco vs. 99.2% SICS, $p = 0.27$).

Open Access This chapter is licensed under the terms of the Creative Commons Attribution-NonCommercial-NoDerivatives 4.0 International License (http://creativecommons.org/licenses/by-nc-nd/4.0/), which permits any non-commercial use, sharing, distribution and reproduction in any medium or format, as long as you give appropriate credit to the original author(s) and the source, provide a link to the Creative Commons license and indicate if you modified the licensed material. You do not have permission under this license to share adapted material derived from this chapter or parts of it.

The images or other third party material in this chapter are included in the chapter's Creative Commons license, unless indicated otherwise in a credit line to the material. If material is not included in the chapter's Creative Commons license and your intended use is not permitted by statutory regulation or exceeds the permitted use, you will need to obtain permission directly from the copyright holder.

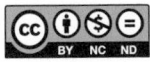

Introduction to Collecting Audit Data

Ralene Sim

Importance of Audit

- Simple and brief quality assurance (QA) audits to ensure key areas reach a minimum standard e.g. annual audit of personal posterior capsular rupture rate in cataract surgery for annual appraisal.
- Quality improvement (QI) audit for new intervention to address problems and gaps (see figure below).

Objectives

- Demonstrating current best practice is in place: High quality, low harm
- Provide evidence that there is good quality of care to patients, regulators such as the Care Quality Commissioning, peers, professional bodies e.g. General Medical Council, The Royal

---

Adapted from: FRCOphth Ophthalmic Services Guidance: Clinical Audit and Clinical Effectiveness in Ophthalmology; October 2016.

R. Sim (✉)
Department of Training and Education, Singapore National Eye Centre, Singapore Eye Research Institute, Singapore, Singapore
e-mail: ralene.sim@mohh.com.sg

College of Ophthalmologists, commissioners, Ministry of Health, World Health Organisation
- Share your outcomes
- Benchmarking for other units, measuring change of standards over time
- Present at conferences and publish in journals:
  - Fulfil appraisal/revalidation
  - Improve quality of care
  - Reduce risk, harm, and clinical mistakes
  - Increase efficiency and effectiveness
  - Direct resources or provide evidence for requirement of resources (e.g. in a business case) for staff, equipment, training

Examples of audit: cataract surgery posterior capsule rupture (PCR) rates, endophthalmitis rates, visual acuity results, and macular hole visual acuity outcomes (Fig. 58.1).

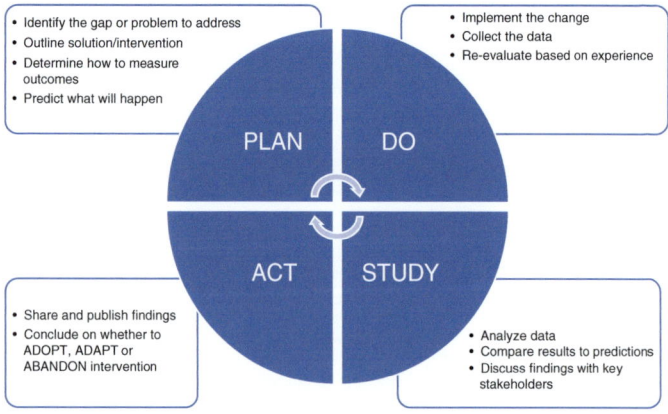

Fig. 58.1 Example of a plan do act study cycle of quality improvement. (Image reproduced with permission and courtesy of SNEC)

GEH Perspectives
1. Frequent audits on common procedures such as cataract surgery and intravitreal injections and strongly encouraged.
2. Important quality data can be used for various reports and publications and can track improvements in response to interventions.
3. The rigour of the audit and the amount of data collected is dependent on the context of the practice, the manpower available and the data management capacity.
4. In line with WHO recommendation, basic data for cataract surgery such as pre- and post-operative visual acuity and severe rates of complications such as endophthalmitis should be prioritized for all services.

Recommended Guidelines for Screening

Eye screening	Age and time frame	Referral criteria
In neonatal period	Neonatal (<4 weeks from birth, preferably within 72 h of birth) or at first encounter with a well-baby clinic (or equivalent); and	Premature infant, low birth weight, unwell or birth defect
	At a postnatal visit, for example at the routine 6-week postnatal check	Significant crust or pus on eyelids
		Eyelid swelling
		Absent/abnormal appearance of eyelashes/eyelids
		Excessive watery or sticky discharge
		Abnormal red on white part of the eye
		Abnormal shape or haziness of coloured part of eye
		Eyes not aligned
		Abnormal/asymmetrical eye movements
		Both eyes different size
		Eyes abnormal in shape or colour
		Red reflex is absent
		If any results abnormal, or unable to be tested, refer for a full eye examination to eye care personnel
Preschool aged children	Aged 3–5 years	Diabetes
		Pain/discomfort/severe itchiness of the eye
		Distance vision worse than 6/12 in either eye

Eye screening	Age and time frame	Referral criteria
School aged children	Aged 5–18 years	Eyelid margin significant crust or pus
		Excessive watery or sticky discharge
		Abnormal red or lesion on white part of eye
	Vision and eye screening conducted every 1–2 years	Abnormal haziness on coloured part of eye
		Eyes are not aligned
		If any results abnormal, or unable to be tested, refer for a full eye examination to eye care personnel
Older adults	Aged 50 years and older	As above +
	Vision and eye screening can be conducted every 1–2 years	Near vision worse than N6 (at distance of 40 cm)
		If no improvement with the trial ready-made spectacles, needs referral

Adapted from WHO—Vision and Eye Screening Implementation Handbook

Open Access This chapter is licensed under the terms of the Creative Commons Attribution-NonCommercial-NoDerivatives 4.0 International License (http://creativecommons.org/licenses/by-nc-nd/4.0/), which permits any non-commercial use, sharing, distribution and reproduction in any medium or format, as long as you give appropriate credit to the original author(s) and the source, provide a link to the Creative Commons license and indicate if you modified the licensed material. You do not have permission under this license to share adapted material derived from this chapter or parts of it.

The images or other third party material in this chapter are included in the chapter's Creative Commons license, unless indicated otherwise in a credit line to the material. If material is not included in the chapter's Creative Commons license and your intended use is not permitted by statutory regulation or exceeds the permitted use, you will need to obtain permission directly from the copyright holder.

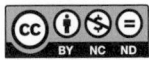

Abbreviations

AC	Anterior Chamber
AMD	Age-Related Macular Degeneration
ANA	Anti-Nuclear Antibodies
ANCA IIF	Antineutrophil Cytoplasmic Antibody Indirect Immunofluorescence
AVP	Anterior Visual Pathway
BP	Blood Pressure
BHIB	Brain Heart Infusion Broth
CL	Contact Lens
CF	Counting Fingers
CMV	Cytomegalovirus
CN	Cranial Nerve
CNS	Central Nervous System
COVID	Coronavirus Disease
CT	Computed Tomography
CRP	C-Reactive Protein
CRVO	Central Retina Vein Occlusion
CSF	Cerebrospinal Fluid
CXR	Chest X-Ray
DM	Diabetes Mellitus
dsDNA	Double-Stranded DNA
ECG	Electrocardiogram
ENA	Extractable Nuclear Antigen
EOM	Extraocular Movement
ESR	Erythrocyte Sedimentation Rate
FB	Foreign Body

FBC	Full Blood Count
EOM	Extra Ocular Movement
GCA	Giant Cell Arteritis
HBA1c	Hemoglobin A1C (glycated haemoglobin)
HIV	Human Immunodeficiency Virus
HZO	Herpes Zoster Ophthalmicus
HTN	Hypertension
HLD	Hyperlipidemia
ICP	Intracranial Pressure
IHD	Ischemic Heart Disease
IF	Immuno-Fluorescence
IM	Intramuscular
IOFB	Intramuscular Foreign Body
IOP	Intra-Ocular Pressure
IVT	Intra-Vitreal Therapy
LPI	Laser Peripheral Iridotomy
MPO	Myelo-Peroxidase
MOG	Myelin Oligonucleotide Glycoprotein
MRA	Magnetic Resonance Angiography
MRI	Magnetic Resonance Imaging
MRV	Magnetic Resonance Venography
NMO	Neuro-Myelitis Optica
NPC	Naso-pharyngeal Carcinoma
NSAID	Non-Steroidal Anti-Inflammatory Drug
OIS	Ocular Ischemic Syndrome
OCT	Optical Coherence Tomography
OT	Operating Theatre
PCR	Polymerase Chain Reaction
PEE	Punctate Epithelial Erosion
PDR	Proliferative Diabetic Retinopathy
PR3	Proteinase 3
PT/aPTT	Prothrombin Time/Activated Partial Thromboplastin Time
PVD	Posterior Vitreous Detachment
RA	Rheumatoid Arthritis
RAPD	Relative Afferent Pupillary Defect
RF	Rheumatoid Factor
RVO	Retina Vein Occlusion

RD	Retina Detachment
SLE	Systemic Lupus Erythematosus
TB	Tuberculosis
VA	Visual Acuity
VDRL	Venereal Disease Research Laboratory
VH	Vitreous Haemorrhage

Annexes

Visual Acuity Check

- Distance visual acuity is commonly assessed using a vision chart at a fixed distance [commonly 6 metres (or 20 feet)].
- The smallest line read on the chart is written as a fraction, where the numerator refers to the distance at which the chart is viewed, and the denominator is the distance at which a "healthy" eye is able to read that line of the vision chart. For example, a visual acuity of 6/18 means that, at 6 metres from the vision chart, a person can read a letter that someone with normal vision would be able to see at 18 metres. "Normal" vision is taken to be 6/6.
- Near visual acuity is measured according to the smallest print size that a person can discern at a given test distance.

Relative Afferent Pupillary Defect (RAPD) Check

- Perform the test in a darkened room.
- Ask the patient to keep looking at a distant fixation target to prevent the near-pupil response (a constriction in pupil size when moving focus from a distant to a near object). While performing the test, take care not to get in the way of the fixation target.
- Swing the whole torch deliberately from one eye to another so that the beam of light is directed directly into each eye.

- Keep the light source at the same distance from each eye to ensure that the light stimulus is equally bright in both.
- Keep the beam of light steadily on the first eye for at least 3 seconds. This allows the pupil size to stabilise.
- Move the light quickly to shine in the other eye. Again, hold the light steady for 3 seconds.
- When the light is shone into the eye with the retinal or optic nerve disease, the pupils of both eyes will constrict, but not fully. This is because of a problem with the afferent pathway.
- When the light is shone into the other, normal (less abnormal) eye, both pupils will constrict further. This is because the afferent pathway of this eye is intact, or less damaged than that of the other eye.
- When the light is shone back into the abnormal eye, both pupils will get larger, even the pupil in the normal eye.
- Positive RAPD: Pupil enlarges after the light is swung from the normal eye into the abnormal eye.

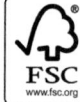

MIX
Papier aus verantwortungsvollen Quellen
Paper from responsible sources
FSC® C105338

If you have any concerns about our products,
you can contact us on
ProductSafety@springernature.com

In case Publisher is established outside the EU,
the EU authorized representative is:
**Springer Nature Customer Service Center GmbH
Europaplatz 3, 69115 Heidelberg, Germany**

Printed by Libri Plureos GmbH
in Hamburg, Germany